I HATE Myself

Overcome Self-Loathing and Realize
Why **You're Wrong About You**

Blaise Aguirre, MD

Foreword by ***JEWEL***

WILEY

Published by John Wiley & Sons, Inc., Hoboken, New Jersey.
Published simultaneously in Canada.

For general information on our other products and services or for technical support, please contact our Customer Care Department within the United States at (800) 762-2974, outside the United States at (317) 572-3993 or fax (317) 572-4002.

Wiley also publishes its books in a variety of electronic formats. Some content that appears in print may not be available in electronic formats. For more information about Wiley products, visit our website at www.wiley.com.

Library of Congress Cataloging-in-Publication Data is Available:

ISBN 9781394299942 (Cloth)
ISBN 9781394299966 (ePDF)
ISBN 9781394299959 (ePub)

Cover Design: Jon Boylan
Cover Images: © Douglas Baldan/Shutterstock, © klyaksun/Shutterstock
Author Photo: Courtesy of Blaise Aguirre

SKY10099108_022825

This book is dedicated to anyone who feels the daily burden of self-hatred. You are deeply loveable. Those who love you know it, and I hope that by the time you have finished the book, you will find your path to defeating self-hatred and recognize that you are so much more than the false narrative that told you that you weren't worth it. You ARE worth it!

Contents

Foreword

When I was 15, I was eating an orange in my hometown of Homer, Alaska. I had eaten an orange many times in my life of course, but this moment was different. My heart was heavy, and I was contemplating moving out on my own, which would entail many responsibilities such as paying rent, electricity, and food bills and of course getting several jobs to cover those costs. But those were details that I could figure out. What was really weighing on me was a problem I did not know how to solve; I was unhappy, and I knew changing where I lived would not actually solve my unhappiness.

For a long time, I thought my dad was "the bad guy." My mom had left home, and my dad soon began drinking and became physically and verbally abusive.

In recent years, I had the realization that even when I was away from my dad, there was still a "bad guy" in my head, and that he came with me everywhere I went. Even then, I knew moving out would not change this. Today, I call it "internalizing my abuser." I had learned how to be so cruel, so unkind, so demeaning in my own inner dialogue, that there were days I could hardly get out of bed. I could not look in a mirror. I was filled with such self-loathing, self-contempt, shame, and worthlessness that being conscious was mostly unbearable. Moving out would not help that. I would bring this "bad guy" with me.

So, there I was, peeling my orange, when I had an "aha!" moment. At the time I had been reading the writings of some Greek philosophers, as well as learning a bit about the impact of nature versus nurture. It got me thinking: what if my nurture was so poor, that I would never get to know my real nature? What if my trauma was so complete, so encompassing, that it might obscure my chance to know the real me? As my fingers dug into the rough and stiff orange peel, the "aha" realization struck. The peel is the orange's way of protecting itself from the outside world. The protective shell has evolved to keep the most valuable parts of the orange, the nourishing fruit and the life-giving seeds, inside. What if I was the same? What if my painful nurture had similarly led me to develop a protective layer in order to keep my true self intact? My nurture, in part, created my personality. My environment led me to make certain assumptions about myself, ones that caused me to develop a specific type of protective defenses.

As a child of abuse and neglect, I made assumptions about my worth and value and I formed a psyche and many personality components around them. For instance, I was mistrustful. I felt worthless. I was suspicious of people. I was always waiting for the world to let me down. I lied or masked to make myself seem more likeable to people. I stole to get my needs met because I believed no one would help me meet them. All of these things formed my "peel." But they were not "me." They were my peel.

I stared at my half-peeled orange, portions of the glistening fruit revealed, and I wondered: *What if the fruit inside was my metaphorical nature, the real me?*

Who was I on the inside? The question stunned me. I had spent my entire life confusing myself for my peel. I spent all my time wrapped up in my thoughts and opinions about myself. I was obsessed with maintaining my hardened exterior, and the assumptions I made about myself. But what if those assumptions were flawed? What if who I was wasn't the mistrustful, self-loathing, worthless person, and the real me existed within me, sweet and nourishing? What if she was just waiting for me to turn my gaze inward to get to know her?

That day changed my life. I realized that for me to move out successfully, I had to develop strategies for what I call *going down and in*. My task was to get beneath my thoughts and my opinions about myself. I had to become intimate with who I was irrespective of my name, my upbringing, my job, my fame, or my family. I learned to go down and in, to fall in love with myself, slowly, and over time. I learned to be patient, compassionate, tender, and curious with, and about, myself. This was particularly hard because I had no model for doing this. No one else had ever shown me such grace, and the process was slow and progressive. To this day, I work on this. I'm still discovering and falling in love with myself. It's rewarding work. It has led to genuine happiness. I can look at my body, my life, my mistakes and feel genuine awe for the human I am.

Once you touch down into the truth of who you are, it makes you powerful. You give yourself something no one can ever take away. You know you. And there is not another one like you.

I hope that in exploring Dr. Aguirre's concepts in this book, you will begin to realize that destructive thoughts and opinions and certainties of self-hatred are not only not true but are distracting you from experiencing the journey of a lifetime – discovering who you actually are. And who you are, I promise, is beautiful. Scars and all.

—Jewel

Grammy-nominated singer-songwriter, humanitarian activist, and mental health advocate

Introduction

Although I have been thinking about this topic for some time, I committed to write this book after a colleague who knew that I was very interested in the topic asked if I would do a consult with a young woman suffering with deep self-loathing. I agreed and when I met the young person, it was clear just how intensely and enduringly she had experienced self-hatred. I told her of my interest in the experience and that I believed that it could change. I asked her if she would be willing to work with me on changing this particular view of herself. To my surprise she said YES.

I say this because in the past, patients have told me that they are willing to work on self-injury, or unhealthy relationships, on emotion regulation, but that self-loathing was immutable and that they did not want to waste their time in therapy working on it.

I told the patient that there were no established protocols for working on self-loathing and that in part we would take the current, though scant, knowledge on the topic and work together to focus on elements that worked and put aside the ones that either felt invalidating or that simply were not helpful.

Since there is limited research specific to self-hate, I don't use an explicit treatment approach, but instead modify techniques from therapies that have proven effective in addressing related issues. I also found that by deeply listening to my patients' experiences, I gleaned valuable insights into what might work, and so I recruited some of them and asked them to collaborate with me in this endeavor. In writing this book, I have brought my patients' own voices in order to capture the totality of their interactions with the feeling of self-hate. My hope was that their first-hand experiences and insights would not only enrich the narrative but also provide valuable perspectives on your own journey from the certainty of self-hatred to one where you can see that you have profound worth. What they shared exceeded all my expectations. Their worth is in their words and their reflections, and I hope that you as a reader will see that you are not alone. You are in a silent community that does not need to be silent nor need to believe the untruths you've believed. You will hear echoes of your own thoughts in their words and then use the exercises and strategies developed as extensions of their experience, as new tools on your path to overcoming self-hatred. As I collected their experiences, I was reminded that even when a patient has largely overcome self-hatred, their self-loathing can still occasionally flair up.

> *"I nearly didn't send this to you because I felt that I could not contribute anything that would be helpful or incremental. The self-hatred assignment was postponed by feelings of self-hatred or at least self-deprecating thoughts."*

This was the response to an email I had sent a patient, someone that I have known for many years, who has done so well in her life and yet who had struggled with self-hatred for many years in her life. I was a little surprised by her response, because she seemed to be doing so much better, with a stable career, a stable group of friends, and optimism about the future, and yet self-hatred remains. It is her experience, and those of so many others, that is the driving force behind this book.

One of the least focused-on experiences in mental health is that of self-loathing. In my career, I have been blessed to see so many people move from the depths of despair to enjoying the little moments of ordinary life. And yet, even for those who are working, or going to school, or are in committed relationships, self-hatred can persist. Tragically, it is an experience that can lead to such despair, that those who are plagued by self-loathing thoughts are at high risk for taking their life. If this is your struggle, it is essential that you know that suicide is not the answer to self-hatred. You were not born with self-hatred and once you realize that you can rewrite many of the false and hurtful conclusions about yourself, you can move from the contemplation of suicide to the embracing of a truer and more aspirational sense of who you are.

The Years Before

> "I do not trust people who don't love themselves and yet tell me, I love you. There is an African saying which is: 'Be careful when a naked person offers you a shirt.'"
>
> —Maya Angelou, The Distinguished Annie Clark Tanner Lecture, 16th-Annual Families Alive Conference, Weber State University, May 8, 1997

In the years before I thought more critically about the problem of self-hatred, I worked with a patient, a senior in high school, who was dedicated to her recovery. She practiced new skills, she did her homework, she came to therapy every week, and slowly she moved from the ravages of emotional suffering to focusing on her academics and applying to college. She took up dance, which she had done as a child, and learned how to play the guitar. Over time she felt more in control of her life and went from seeing me twice a week to once a week and then once every two weeks. I noticed, though, that whenever she did something that she perceived as wrong or imperfect, that she would become extremely critical of herself.

"I hate myself," she said one day.

"That's a bit harsh," I said, "everyone makes mistakes."

She looked at me with what I interpreted as confusion, and maybe even some scorn.

"You really don't get it. I hate myself. This is not about making mistakes. Yes, making mistakes highlights what a terrible person I am, but I hate myself now and I have always hated myself," she said.

"But what about all the things that you are doing with your life. Your grades, your college applications, your guitar, your dance?" I persisted.

"Those things make me competent. They don't make me love myself," she said definitively.

"I never knew this about you. Can you tell me more? What a terrible way to see yourself. How can you possibly imagine that you are so awful?"

She sat back and said: "Have a look at my life. I have ruined it. I have ruined the relationships that I care about. I probably ruin your life, too.

Do you know why my parents are divorced? Me. Do you know why my boyfriend left me, and why I will never have a boyfriend again? Me. Do you see my scars? Do you know who made them? Me. Do you know why my mom is constantly worried sick? Me. Do you think she wants to spend six hours per week getting me back and forth to therapy? Do you think that she has nothing better to do with her time? It's because of me. I poison everything I touch, because I am toxic, and the world would be better off without me, such a toxic person."

It saddened me that someone I thought so highly of, thought so poorly of herself. She insisted that she was pure loathing and that there was nothing endearing about her whatsoever.

Despite her gains, this self-perspective did not budge, and in fact, my attempts to get her to see that she had good and love in her, increasingly felt invalidating.

"No matter how much you try to convince me otherwise, there is no good in me. It makes me think that you don't really know me, and that therapy is a waste of time. You are confusing my hard work at being more effective and less suicidal, with me caring about myself more. False, I just want to be able to make it through the day. Let's just focus on me being more effective."

She continued to make great strides, got into her top choice of college though early action, was dancing regularly and had made some friends at school. The topic of her self-loathing was left unaddressed, because she thought it was futile and that my bringing it up was invalidating. Also, I didn't know what to do and how to budge the debilitating and toxic symptom.

That Christmas, she came for session, and brought me a Christmas card. She had spent some weeks working on it, and the level of artistic precision, attention to color detail, and word sentiment, captured a devotion and dedication that I rarely find.

"Thank you," I said. "You have gone to a lot of trouble to make it. It is beautiful and your words mean so much to me. You say so many nice things. Why did you make it?"

"You have helped me so much, and I appreciate it. I just wanted to show you how much it meant to me," she said smiling.

"But I am confused, because what you write almost implies, that you care about me," I said with intention. "I am sorry to say that I cannot accept your card. I cannot accept a lie."

Her smile turned to shock. "What do you mean? Of course I care about you."

"But caring is a form of love," I persisted.

"So?" She seemed confused.

I asked, "Well how can you give me something that is not yours to give. If you steal $100 from someone, it is not yours to give to me. You can only authentically give me something that is truly yours to give. Otherwise, it is a lie. You give me a card that shows caring for me and gratitude for me, but you cannot give caring and love that you don't have, and so you giving me those things is a lie, and I have to reject your card, but appreciate the effort."

She was defeated and started to cry. "I can't believe it. It took me such a long time to make the card, and I did it because I care about you, and you reject it???"

"Wait," I said, "are you saying that you do have caring inside you?"

"Yes, of course I do!"

I said, "But you have spent so many months telling me that you had no love in you, that you were a toxic person, that you poisoned everyone you met! I am beyond overjoyed by what you are telling me! Of course, if your card comes from love and caring I can accept it and joyfully so! But here is the thing, if you have love inside of you, you are not all the things that you say about yourself, and if you have love and compassion for me, it is in you, and you can start to see that. It is in you. And if it is in you, it is in you for yourself. And if you have love inside of you, how can you be so toxic? Your card would only have poisoned me if it were evil, but it comes from kindness."

Over the next few months, she started to notice moments of acts of kindness and compassion to others and recognized that these acts came from a place of genuine caring, from deep within. And that her caring, and compassion had to be within, and that if it was within herself for others, it was within herself for herself. With time, self-loathing eroded until all that was left was a sadness for the young girl who had not known to love herself. This was an important first for me, and a fundamentally important experience for my patient. Self-loathing had shifted.

Unchangeable?

> "Every single thing I touch becomes sick with sadness, 'cause it's all over now, all out to sea."
>
> —Taylor Swift, from "Bigger Than The Whole Sky"

For people with conditions like borderline personality disorder, also known as BPD, a condition that I review in a later chapter, the experience of self-hatred does not feel as if is something that can change. It does not feel like a perspective. It has the quality of being core to who they are. When I ask those who feel this way if they have addressed it in therapy, I receive three main comments:

1. No, no one ever asked me about it.
2. Yes, I brought it up once, but they simply told me to practice self-compassion.
3. No, I never thought about bringing it up because it IS who I am and although I can change many of my behaviors, I can't change who I am.

When I hear these comments, I feel profound sadness because the people making these statements are supremely talented and compassionate to others, and when I get to know them over years of therapy, I feel deep caring for them. How is it possible that someone so loveable feels so unlovable?

I want to be as clear as I can be on my perspectives on self-hatred. It is a pathological state. It is a source of enduring suffering, and one that blinds you from seeing your true self, and all that is good in you. It can end up destroying your mind and tragically it can lead you down the path to suicidal thinking. In these pages, I hope to convince you that self-hatred is a deception created by a mind that learned to hate itself, and that you can learn its opposite, that you are worthy.

Structure of the Book

For the purposes of this book, I use the terms *self-hatred* and *self-loathing* interchangeably. This is because most of my patients tell me that they are the same thing. Throughout the book, I weave narrative, dialogue, and reflections with research. Some of the ideas may feel familiar and validating, and some of it may feel too scientific. The science is important as all of therapy, all of what works, must be based in ideas and practices that can be replicated and practiced by others in different contexts. When it comes to research on self-hatred, there is not a lot, and I think that this has to do with the fact that few patients present for therapy with self-hatred as a primary complaint, and also that mental health professionals don't ask about it in their evaluations.

I don't think that this is a book that you necessarily need to read cover to cover. If the science feels too tedious, I have indicated the sections that you can skip without losing the thread of the helpful points.

In the book I have assigned exercises that my patients have told me were helpful to them. There are lined spaces for your answers below each exercise. I have used analogies and metaphors to try to explain what certain concepts mean. Finally, over the years, I have collected quotes about the experience of self-loathing reflected by poets, novelists, philosophers, athletes, and musicians. I have peppered these throughout the book: They underscore that the experience is far more universal than only in people who come for therapy.

I hope you find this useful in your journey to overcoming self-loathing and that each reader with lived experience can one day see how essential and loveable they are. Know that your value is not defined by the way you were treated, your perceived flaws, mistakes you have made, or what others say about you. You are no different from anyone else who is inherently worthy of being loved, and if you are skeptical, read on and let me, and all the contributors to this book, accompany you on a journey to seeing yourself as a person of worth and value.

Part 1

Understanding Self-Hatred

Chapter 1

What Is Self-Hatred?

"Why does shame and self-loathing become cruelty to the innocent?"
—Anne Rice, *Merrick*

Self-hatred is not a choice. You are not presented with the options of loving yourself or hating yourself and choose to hate yourself. Self-hatred is there because you were led to believe that it is true. Your early experiences were not your fault. Any bad thing that happened to you was not because you decided that it was what you wanted. Experience after experience led you to believe that you were not worthy. You did not make self-hatred happen, and self-hatred does not have to be what endures. You have the power within you to define and validate your experience and then change something that you believe would never change.

I recently decided to re-read *Jane Eyre* by Charlotte Brontë written in 1847. 1847 was a time decades before we understood the impact of trauma and invalidation on a person's sense of self. Reading the book through the lens of my current exploration, I was shocked to see how profoundly Brontë understood and articulated this impact. For instance, here is her protagonist, Jane, describing an experience at 10 years old:

> *Mrs. Reed soon rallied her spirits: she shook me most soundly, she boxed both my ears, and then left me without a word. Bessie supplied the hiatus by a homily of an hour's length, in which she proved beyond a doubt that I was the most wicked and abandoned child ever reared under a roof. I half believed her; for I felt indeed only bad feelings surging in my breast."*
>
> *—Jane Eyre by Charlotte Brontë*

The experience of many patients is reflected in this passage and you can have deep compassion for the 10-year-old Jane because you see that she did not choose to be treated in such a hurtful way. And then through years of being treated this way, it makes sense that she concludes that it must be because she is such a terrible child.

Self-hatred is a lie that arises from experiences that you had no way of preventing. In many cases you were too little.

The self-hatred that I tackle in this book is not some transient state. For the people with lived experience, it is a persistent, unrelenting and unyielding intense dislike of the self, and one that comes with feelings of inadequacy, guilt, self-blame, and low self-worth. People with self-hatred at times see themselves as a burden that needs to be removed from the world. There is an enduring sense that "I will never be good enough."

Not Just Messing Up

This core self-hatred is not transient. It is not the same as, for example, someone accidently spilling a glass of red wine on a white tablecloth, or breaking a plate, or messing up on a term paper, saying: "I'm so stupid, I hate myself." Many people have said "I hate myself" to express dissatisfaction in an outcome or an action. In this context, it typically means that they messed up; they use the expression to acknowledge to themselves and others that they are aware of messing up. "I hate myself," uttered in these types of situations is a transient reflection of temporary upset.

50 Shades of Reaction

There are degrees of reaction when an accident happens, such as spilling red wine on a white tablecloth. For those who do not suffer from self-hate, there may be a moment of surprise or embarrassment, followed by an apology to their host, and an offer to clean up or to pay for a new tablecloth. Then, after the wine-spilling (or whatever incident) and apology, they continue enjoying their time without dwelling on the incident. In contrast, for those who suffer from self-hate, the reaction is quite different. Intense feelings of shame and guilt emerge, their inner dialogue becomes harsh and critical, and they experience deep embarrassment, guilt, or even self-disgust. They struggle to move past the incident, which weighs on their mind for the remainder of the day. While to many, it is just spilled wine; to those with self-hate, it is a reflection of their own perceived inadequacies.

So you will see, self-loathing I discuss in this book is a much deeper, painful, and all-consuming problem. It is a construct that evolves over time and seems to become embedded in the very essence of the person as a core part of the self. It is as if self and self-hatred have merged and cannot be separated, to the point that a person can never remember not hating themselves, or that the idea of challenging it seems preposterous, even a waste of time. *"Self-hatred is to me what H2 is to O in water. Water is H2O. That's me and self-hatred,"* quipped a patient.

For most people, self-hatred and self-loathing are the same thing, and I tend to use the term interchangeably throughout the book; however, one patient felt differently. She felt that self-loathing was even more intense than self-hatred and said:

> *It's loud in my head, all the time. So much of it is me berating my own existence. Everything I do is wrong. Nothing I do is good enough. Maybe the little failures of each day seem like nothing to other people, but when my head is already SCREAMING at me that I can't do anything right, even forgetting to put grape jelly on my daughter's PB&J instead of strawberry feels like the end of the world. How can I not mess even the little stuff up?! Sure, maybe I'm a nobody that can't figure out how to make it in this world, but AT LEAST I could put the right fucking jelly on the sandwich.*
>
> *"Except I can't."*
>
> *"That's self-loathing right there. Hatred is a walk in the park next to self-loathing. Self-loathing is the peak of the mountain of self-hatred."*

"That's kinda funny and clever!" I said, "Can't you have some admiration for a mind that came up with that?"

"No, because only a mind that hates itself would come up with that. I wish that I had never had to think that" she replied solemnly.

"Well," I reflected, "you are so much more than hydrogen and oxygen and so maybe if you can also see all the other things that make you up, your focus on this one idea might change."

She shrugged skeptically.

I asked a patient to express the idea in a way that others might get it, and she said: *"I would describe my self-loathing to others as a pervasive feeling of being a bad person with no sense of worth or identity. And I mean ALL the time. I often feel that I am a disgusting person who is at fault for all of the problems in my life and who does not deserve care, compassion, or good things generally. And I mean ALL the time. In addition, I feel a sense of separation from self and like it does not matter if I like myself because I don't have a sense of self-concept and often don't feel grounded in reality."*

Many people who live this way, feel that they are so flawed that they must, by virtue of these flaws, be punished for their very existence. And another point is that it endures. "People who have headaches don't know what unrelenting migraines are," explained a patient who suffers from migraines and borderline personality disorder (BPD).

At times, self-destructive and self-degrading behavior follows as an attempt to self-punish. Self-destructive and self-degrading behavior used as self-punishment never works, even if there is some temporary relief. It doesn't work for various reasons; firstly, punishment is typically used when a person has done something wrong or committed a crime. What is it that you need to be punished for? There never was a crime for which you deserved punishment to begin with. If you were abused as a child, a crime was committed, but not by you. Secondly, the very "punishment" behaviors you inflict on yourself often leave you feeling even worse about yourself than when you started. And, finally, even if you had committed some crime, once you've been punished for the crime, you've served your time, and no further punishment is required. Why keep punishing yourself? Think of a person going to jail for robbing a bank; after the person is released, they don't keep going to jail for the same crime.

When a person is feeling strong self-hatred, they not only feel that they don't deserve the love of others, but they also feel that they don't deserve anything good happening to them, and instead conclude that anything bad that happens is, to them, a manifestation of their awfulness, and a deserved punishment for being such a terrible person.

I was once working with a patient who arrived a few minutes late. She said: "Now do you see what a terrible human being I am? I mean I wasted your time. That's what I do and that's what I am, a terrible waste of time and a terrible waste of humanity."

"Wow, that's harsh. I was looking forward to our session," I said. "You are always on time and so I was a little bit worried, but you're only 10 minutes late. I assume that you hit traffic, or that you woke up late, or that you were talking to your girlfriend, or that something came up at work. I never even considered that my time was being wasted. And to be honest, I quickly finished an email that I had forgotten to send. Not only am I not at all upset. It wouldn't even come into my mind. In fact, I am grateful I was able to send the email. I appreciate the extra few minutes!"

"Why are you being nice?" she asked. "I deserve to be punished for being a terrible, horrible patient. You should not be thanking me. There are no excuses for being late. I want to punish myself, but you should punish me instead. If you came over and slapped me, then it would make sense."

I think that I started to tear up, because she said, "What's wrong?"

"It just saddens me that you hate yourself so much, that you imagine that I hate you so much that you deserve to be punished for something that happens millions of times a day, to millions of people because of the circumstances of their lives, and then that you would be surprised that in fact I have no such feelings of malice or contempt for you. I know that you are doing the best that you can." I stopped to reflect. "For many people who hate themselves, they cannot imagine that others don't see them in the way that they see themselves. You hate yourself, and you imagine, or maybe believe, that I and others who care about you, can't possibly care about you. You worry that they are lying to you, or that they are deluded or that they cannot see how terrible you are. A psychodynamic therapist would say that you project your self-hatred onto

others and then believe that projection that they hate you. In a way, by being so certain about what they believe and how they should treat you, you rob them of an opportunity to have their own experience of you. In my case, I admire the very hard work in your efforts to overcome the mental health obstacles to you getting into college. And that admiration is true whether you believe it to be so or not. You telling me that I am wrong, is like saying that I am not allowed to have an opinion other than yours on this."

"You see, I 'rob' you of your experience, I am not terrible?" she countered.

"You are a terrible knower of what I think," I said smiling, and the tensions diffused.

Related Concepts

Colleagues have suggested that when I focus on self-hatred as a separate entity, that what I am discussing is a set of ideas that is common in many psychiatric conditions, and that many people with other mental health conditions are discontent with themselves and with how their brains work. However, my experience tells me that self-hate can manifest in two distinct ways: firstly, as a symptom of underlying mental health conditions AND secondly, as a standalone experience, one that lingers even when the fury of other mental health conditions has done its worst. It has me thinking: Could enduring self-hatred, in the absence of other clinical symptoms, be its own diagnosis?

When I ask my patients with self-loathing if self-hatred is simply part of a mental health condition, they acknowledge that they identify with all of the ideas that we are shortly about to review, but that they are not the same. They say that self-loathing includes many or all of the following experiences but that having any one of these related concepts would be far easier to deal with and would be far less impactful, less all-encompassing, and less painful than self-loathing. "If all it was, was self-criticism, I would not want to die so badly," was the reflection of one of my patients.

Many people with enduring self-loathing express the following phrases: "I'm a failure," "I can't do anything right," "no one is ever going to like me," "I will never be good enough," "I'll never get better," "I deserve to suffer because I am such a terrible person," "I should just die," "I deserve to be punished," "I should never be in a relationship because I am toxic to others," "I am to blame for all my problems and those of other people," "everyone hates me." Certainly, these don't help reduce the impact of self-hatred.

Let's have a deeper look at concepts related to self-hatred and see how they are similar and how they are different. For some readers of this book, the concepts may in fact mean the same thing as self-hatred, and yet for others, they are ideas that don't resonate. Some of these concepts have a research base and are clinically defined, whereas other concepts are the words that those with lived experience have used.

Concepts and Experiences Related to, but Different from, Self-Loathing

Self-Criticism

> "If you're capable of despising your own behavior, you might just love yourself."
>
> —Criss Jami

Self-criticism is the tendency to engage in, and with, negative self-evaluation leading to feelings of worthlessness, feeling that you are a failure, and feeling guilty when you don't meet expectations. Self-criticism was originally seen as particularly relevant to the development of a specific type of depression, known as introjective depression. In clinical practice, we no longer use that term; however, it is useful to think about because historical descriptions of patients with this type of depression seem to be consistent with many of the themes in this book. Therapists would notice that some patients with introjective depression would feel deserving of being punished and so interpret therapists' comments as punishing.

When seen as a personality trait, research finds that self-criticism has been linked to several negative consequences. In a study examining behavior differences between people who were self-critical and those who weren't

(Mongrain 1998), the research found that self-critics experienced greater negative mood states, perceived that others were not trying to help, and made fewer requests for help. Interestingly, in their study, they found that those with and without self-criticism did not actually differ in the amount of support they received, but rather, in how they perceived the support they got, in how they accepted it, and how frequently they asked for help.

In another study (Santor et al. 2000), in people who were self-critical, when compared with those who were not self-critical, the self-criticism predicted a decrease in agreeable or kind comments toward their partners and also predicted being more blaming of their partners than those who were not self-critical. As you can see, this is not exactly the same as self-hatred although there may be some elements that are similar.

I asked a patient about his experience of self-criticism, and this was his reflection: *"I've always been extremely self-critical.... So, does that mean that it is part of my personality? It's different from my self-hatred. Do you think that it could be stemming from my other mental health struggles [like could it be part of my OCD or pathological perfectionism] or is it a separate issue? Either way, that makes self-loathing harder to treat because self-criticism is so deeply ingrained in my way of thinking and acting."*

Another patient said: *"No. These are two different ideas. You can be criticizing of certain aspects of yourself/things you've done without despising every aspect of yourself."*

The bottom line is that while many people who hate themselves experience self-criticism, most people who criticize themselves, do not also hate themselves.

Self-Disgust

According to research (Overton et al. 2008), self-disgust is a negative self-conscious emotional pattern of thinking that organizes and interprets incoming information. Self-disgust originates from the basic emotion of disgust and is directed toward physical self, meaning physical self-disgust, and accompanied by statements like: "I find myself repulsive" or to some aspects of your behavior, behavioral self-disgust, with statements like: "I often do things I find revolting."

Research (Ypsilanti et al. 2020) shows that self-disgust has been associated with many psychological difficulties, including social anxiety, impaired body image, disordered eating behavior, and PTSD symptoms in women with a history of sexual assault. When these researchers looked at self-disgust in military veterans, they found that veterans with PTSD reported almost three times higher scores in self-disgust, and significantly higher scores in loneliness, anxiety, and depression, when compared to the general population, and that it was the self-disgust that connected the experiences of loneliness and anxiety. In this group, loneliness was defined as the subjective experience of lack of meaningful social relationships, which is common among war veterans.

I find it interesting that when I ask most of the patients who endure self-loathing about self-disgust, that self-disgust does not resonate as strongly as self-hatred. Many feel that it is a different thing. One patient who experienced both self-loathing and self-disgust told me: *"I always hate myself, but I don't always feel self-disgust. When I do have self-disgust, it makes my self-loathing worse. God forbid that I walk by a mirror, and I see my reflection. Then I am disgusted by the person looking back at me. I was shopping at the mall with a friend, and he was checking himself out every time we walked by a shop window. I looked the other way. But now that you asked the question, there is another way that self-disgust shows up. You know like when you step in dogshit you are disgusted and want to wash it off as quickly as you can? Well, sometimes if I am at a party and I use the rest room and wash my hands and see myself, my self-disgust shows up. When I go back into the party, I feel that I am like that dogshit, and I think: 'My being in this room makes me think that they are probably thinking that there is something horrible and disgusting in the room, and that thing is me. My leaving would be the best thing I could do for them.'"*

Another patient also recognized that there was stronger overlap with self-disgust than with other ideas: *"This is the closest (in my opinion) to self-loathing, if not, the same. I can't think of anything to differentiate the two."*

"And I saw my reflection in a lake, and I waited for it to freeze a little bit so I could break it with my boot."

—Sam Pink

Another patient had a different, and somewhat comical, take on self-disgust: *"Self-disgust, for me, is PART of self-loathing. I love the dictionary definition. Revulsion. No doubt, I am repulsed by every aspect of my being. I do think it's possible to be disgusted with yourself yet not hate or loathe yourself, though. Humans are really disgusting creatures, but their disgustingness isn't necessarily bad. Am I disgusted by the amount of farting that comes out of my husband? Absolutely. I certainly don't hate or loathe him for it. I guess it turns into hatred or loathing when it becomes a choice."*

To underscore this point, I have an acquaintance who is significantly overweight. At social outings he eats a lot of high-calorie foods. He is an open, friendly, and well-liked person, and he is a self-described "bon-vivant." He lives a life of consumption and tells me he's the very definition of a hedonist. I once asked him if he had any regrets about his excesses. *"Only when I walk by a mirror or go clothes shopping," he answered, "when I see myself I kinda gross myself out. I'm really kinda disgusted by myself, but I don't spend too much time thinking about it. I mean that would take the pleasure out of EVERYTHING!"*

It makes sense that the concepts of self-disgust and self-hatred are related and connected; however, research and clinical experience defines them as different constructs.

EXERCISE

Do you experience self-disgust? Y/N

If so, how would you describe the experience to others?

____

____

____

____

Self-Blame

Self-blame is the act of attributing the consequences of an experience to be the direct result of your actions or your character. It is related to the concept of the perception of control, and people who blame themselves a lot are more likely to believe they have greater control over their lives than those who don't. In researching the concept of self-blame, I found it curious that many of the research articles had to do with medical conditions and the blaming of the self as a reason why the person developed the medical conditions. The articles had titles like:

> *"Self-blame attributions in women with newly diagnosed breast cancer: A prospective study of psychological adjustment."*
> *(Glinder and Compas* 1999*)*

> *"The role of self-blame and responsibility in adjustment to inflammatory bowel disease."*
> *(Voth and Sirois* 2009*)*

> *"Smoking and drinking behavior in patients with head and neck cancer: Effects of behavioral self-blame and perceived control."*
> *(Christensen et al.* 1999*)*

There are of course many psychological conditions and experiences where people blame themselves and that can happen when people have experienced trauma. This is especially true even when the traumatic event was never of your making at all: You didn't ask for it, you weren't okay with it happening, you didn't go out looking for it and yet you were traumatized. There are cultures where society blames the victim for the trauma. "Oh, if she had only not dressed that way," or "He should not have been at that party," or "She should not have been drinking," and so on. The vast majority of people dress in certain ways, go to certain parties, and have a drink and they are okay. Nothing bad happens to them. They don't go into situations looking to be traumatized. And yet, if a traumatic experience happens, many end up blaming themselves. There are many reasons why you might blame yourself, whether it's a single event or prolonged childhood trauma.

Here are some ideas to consider:

If you were traumatized as a child, your perspective as an adult is different than what it was when you were a child. What was that child's point of view? Remember children don't have the developmental capacity and perspective to see the flaws and wounds and deficits of the people who were supposed to be taking care of them. Because children don't have this capacity, they conclude that they must have been to blame for what happened to them.

For some children and even adults, self-blame can serve as a type of protection because the idea of blaming the very person or people who were supposed to be on their side can destroy the perception that they are always going to be there, to provide and care for them. "If I blame them, then they are the ones who abused me, so I can't trust them and so I shouldn't be with them. But then I will be all alone in the world, and that is even more unbearable." This can feel even more true if you were the focus of the trauma and your siblings or friends were spared from abuse.

An interesting twist on the perception of self-control is that for people who believe that they have a lot of control, when things go well, there is a sense of well-being. In 1979, researchers (Janoff-Bulman) proposed two types of self-blame: The first was one that was adaptive, where the person's sense of control-oriented response was focused on the person's behavior. For example, say a person has set a goal of trying to walk two miles every day and one day they don't make it. They tell themselves that they have to try harder, maybe wake up earlier and not have so many items on their schedule. In this sense, their behavior is under their control, and they are then to blame if they succeed or not. This type of self-control and self-responsibility may be considered healthier, but it is not always the case if the person feels that every single outcome in their lives is based on trying harder. In these cases, it tends to bump into the second and more maladaptive type of self-blame where the focus is on esteem-oriented response, on the person's character. In this example, the person might then say, "I am to blame for not having completed the two miles because I am a lazy and unmotivated person."

Now, although many people with self-hatred often blame themselves when things go wrong, not everyone who blames themselves hates themselves. They may feel responsible for negative outcomes, but this is not typically because they hate themselves. They can point to some other negative self-attribution such as that something negative happened because: I am lazy, I am inattentive, I am unmotivated, I am uncaring, and so on. It is not typical that someone who blames themselves for a negative outcome feels that self-hatred is the reason for the negative outcome.

I asked a patient if self-hatred and self-blame were the same. She said: *"No. You can blame yourself for something specifically, without despising every aspect of yourself."*

EXERCISE

a. Do you blame yourself when something you try doesn't work out or has a negative outcome? Y/N

What is an example of this?

____

____

b. Do you blame yourself because of the behavior or actions you took? Y/N

If so, what behavior do you feel that you need to change in order to have better outcomes?

____

____

c. Do you blame yourself because of some perceived character flaw? Y/N

If so, what are the character flaws that you believe cause negative outcomes in whatever you try?

____

____

d. If you experience self-hatred, do you also experience self-blame? Y/N

How are the two tied together for you?

____

____

____

Self-Contempt

> "My ideal date would involve painful silence. My ideal date wouldn't involve me."
>
> —Sam Pink

Many people use the concept of self-contempt as synonymous with self-loathing, and yet is it the same thing? A group of researchers (Beuchat et al. 2023) noted that self-contempt "is a frequent but overlooked clinical phenomenon, associated with a number of psychological problems such as increased sadness and shame." They noted that self-contempt interferes with emotional processing and the quality of the alliance with therapists. However, they noted that there was no clear definition of what self-contempt is.

In their research, they studied a group of 61 participants who were divided into three groups: 20 controls, 21 patients with a diagnosis of BPD and 20 patients with a diagnosis of major depressive disorder. They started with considering self-contempt as a form of anger and scorn toward the self, one that fiercely rejects the self and that is marked by emotional coldness and aloofness.

Already we start to see a difference between self-contempt and self-loathing. Self-contempt has an active, rejecting, and scornful quality to it.

It is as if the person has contempt for a self that almost seems alien. For people with self-loathing, this is not a familiar experience, and that is because it feels as if the loathing is part of them.

ANALOGY: Think of it this way. Say a person does not like the shape of their nose. A person with self-loathing would accept that their nose is a part of them, believe that they deserve it and feel that is just a manifestation of who they are. The person with self-contempt would have contempt for their nose, reject it, and be angry that they have it.

Other researchers (Rüsch et al. 2019) linked self-contempt to what they term "self-stigma." In their study of 77 people, they noted that people with mental illness often internalize public prejudice and negative emotional reactions to their group, and that this leads to self-contempt. The researchers assessed self-contempt, depressive symptoms, hopelessness, and suicidality at the start of the study, and then again three months later. They found that high self-contempt at the initial assessment predicted increased suicidality at three months, and they concluded that self-contempt could be a risk factor for suicidality and recommended that part of mental health interventions should include the targeting of self-stigma and its emotional consequences.

This resonates with the reflection of a patient: *"It's somewhat ironic that having a mental illness only validates the feelings of (for simplicity's sake) self-hatred. Maybe it stems from trauma, or invalidation, or a crazy parent.... WHATEVER. But the deeper we get into our mental illness, the more we're told that we're crazy, that we aren't good enough, that we're a burden, that we aren't trying hard enough, that we're choosing to be this way, that we haven't seen enough doctors or therapists, that we haven't sampled enough drugs or utilized enough skills, that we've caused bankruptcy, that our in-laws hate us, that we're just making things worse for ourselves. And when you live in a world that is swirling with examples of how you've effectively fucked everything up, that there's no going back, there's no fixing it, the damage is done – you tend to hate yourself even more. You feel that stigma and then you stigmatize yourself."*

The bottom line is that although self-contempt is conceptually different from self-loathing, it does seem to share the attribute that it puts the person who experiences it at higher risk for suicide. As the researchers in the few articles on self-loathing and related topics conclude, we have to do more research on including the reduction of these symptoms as a key component to overall recovery.

EXERCISE

Do you experience self-contempt? Y/N

If so, how would you describe the experience to others, and how does it differ from self-blame and self-disgust?

____

____

____

____

It is true that many people with self-loathing feel worthless and feel hopeless, but most do not meet clinical criteria for major depression, and even in the cases when they do and the depression is treated, the self-loathing does not respond to the treatment of depression. Medication does not treat self-hatred.

Perhaps as you read the comments of others, their words will resonate, and if you are stuck in the persistence of self-loathing, these courageous people who shared their words did so to acknowledge their experience and as a first step in facing this toxic false narrative. They are all in various stages of seeing that they and self-hatred are not one, and this for some has brought increasing moments of relief and joy. Some have also noted sadness when something they believed could never change, has started to change, and this is paired with the thought, "why have I suffered so long with this false certainty."

All the Related Concepts

When I asked a patient about these related comments, she reflected on the question and said this the following day: *"I would conceptualize self-criticism, self-blame, and self-disgust more as symptoms of the self-loathing rather than as the loathing itself. I think that another important aspect of self-loathing is self-targeted rage. My self-loathing is a combination of all of these things, with the addition of a background feeling of a lack of sense of identity and only finding identity in the idea in the self-criticism, self-blame, self-disgust, and self-targeted rage."*

Clearly, for many people these related concepts resonate but they are not the same thing. They seem to be some of the ingredients of a larger concept; that is, self-hatred, but they are not self-hatred itself.

An Eastern Point of View

Is self-loathing a Western construct?

Some of the ideas in this section may sound strange or even stressful to consider; however, I cannot profess to have considered a broad set of ideas on the topic of self-loathing without looking at it from all angles, including the perspective of Eastern religion and psychology. If you want to skip this section, you can. I include it because almost all the research in this book has been done in the West, and I recognize that this book is Western-centric.

In reading *Ethics for the New Millennium* (1999) by the Dalai Lama, I was fascinated by his surprise in encountering the idea of self-hatred and self-loathing in conversations with his Western followers. He found the notion "incoherent." He explains his view, reflecting that the very idea of self-loathing is problematic because he believes that all people want to be happy and want to avoid suffering, and so the idea of regarding oneself as worthless seems to contradict the fundamental principles which serve self-interest. Essentially, if you want to be happy and you don't want to suffer, why would you want to hate yourself? The Dalai Lama's thinking on this changed after consultation with Western psychologists, and he then recognized that self-contempt was possible, but concluded that it develops as a basic error of self-evaluation. He suggested that people who hated themselves had lost "all sense of perspective" and developed a "narrowing of vision," which then led to despair.

Clearly the Dalai Lama is not a psychologist with an understanding of the impact of early childhood adversity and maltreatment on the development of self-loathing. Again, in the service of being comprehensive, I include a review of certain forms of Eastern religious philosophy.

In Buddhist teaching, there is an instruction that in addition to giving up thinking too well of oneself one must abandon thinking too badly of oneself. In this philosophy, self-contempt is defined as what is described as the conceited idea, "I am inferior." This conceit involves a powerful sense that the person is inferior to everyone. The teachings describe an excessive form of inferiority known as "self-abasement," where the person asserts that they are even more inferior than the most inferior person, which comes across as arrogant.

So how is it that Buddhist philosophy considers self-loathing to be a type of pride or conceit, rather than, as Western psychologies regard it, the opposite? It is because Buddhist teachings state that the conceit of inferiority, that is the thinking that you are the worst of the worst, is like any form of pride that elevates you above others and is a form of self-affirmation. In this context, the theory is that by highlighting that a person is worse than everyone else, that this attestation is a form of drawing attention to oneself, "Look at me. I am the worst person ever."

Although this is not the experience of my patients, it is nevertheless an interesting point of view, particularly if a person clings to the idea that they have to be worse than everyone else and that because of this they deserve more scorn and hatred than others.

However you got to the belief of self-hatred, remind yourself that from the minute that you, and any one of us was able to explore the world, we did so because we are human and born with an innate sense of curiosity. When this curiosity, shaped by our temperament and biology, interacts with countless situations we encounter, it cultivates the potential to bring our uniqueness and wonder to the world.

But all of this potential can be derailed when the seeds of self-hatred are sown into a young, naïve, and all-accepting mind. These seeds are created by the interaction between a self that is highly sensitive and an environment that is rejecting, invalidating, and hurtful. These seeds then grow into a destructive force that can permeate all your future thoughts, emotions, and behaviors.

And so, when a child repeatedly receives the message that they are not good enough, it becomes their truth. Then, during their childhood and adolescence, as their sense of who they are is evolving, every critical, belittling, abusive, or devaluing interaction leads them to conclude that "if others see me this way, it must be true."

When the external criticisms become internalized, it leads to a fusion of the external and the internal. Self-hatred becomes "who I am," rather than "what I experienced or what I was taught." Self-hatred takes root and becomes further reinforced by an unrelenting inner monologue that has either filtered out or discounted all positive experiences. Instead, the self-hate narrative is accepted or only the negative thoughts are allowed in. Given this continuous negative dialogue, it is completely understandable that you came to the conclusion of self-hatred. There was little that your younger brain could have done.

While your younger self had limited agency in this process, you now have the power to erode, and eventually dismantle, the toxic building blocks that led to such a hurtful core self-belief. In the next chapter, I'll review why it is so critical that you tackle self-hatred.

Chapter 2

Why Is Overcoming Self-Hatred So Critical?

"If you had a person in your life treating you the way you treat yourself, you would have gotten rid of them a long time ago...."

—Cheri Huber

Many people who experience self-hatred, also face other aversive situations. For instance, there are the fears of abandonment, of rejection, of being judged. There is exposure to maltreatment and abuse. There can be self-destructive behaviors. When there are so many issues and concerns in a person's life, why single out self-hatred?

There are two major reasons why:

a. For people with lived-experience, those with self-hatred suffer tremendously because of it, and typically, they have nowhere to talk about it. Even if they are in therapy, it is almost never addressed in therapy.

b. The small amount of research that exists appears to indicate that it is a very strong risk factor for the contemplation of, and acting on, and completion of suicide.

A) The Suffering It Causes: Lived Experience

When a person goes to a doctor or some other mental health specialist, it is common practice for the clinician to want to know a few things:

1. What brings you to therapy?
2. What are your concerns?
3. How has your life been impacted by your symptoms?

If, for example, a person's anxiety is so crippling that they cannot work, or their depression so debilitating that they cannot take care of themselves or their relationships, then working on anxiety and depression would be an essential part of treatment because these are significantly interfering with a person's quality of life.

What about self-loathing? Does it similarly impact a person's experience of life, their aspirations, sense of self and relationships? Is it that bad? Should we in the mental health profession be paying closer attention to the experience? I turned to my experts with lived experience to help me with this question, and this is what they said:

Answer 1: *"It's really hard to even think of a friendship/relationship where I have felt totally secure because of constantly hating myself for everything that I think is wrong about me. My goals in school and life in general are always impeded by self-loathing thoughts. Every single time I've ever had a job interview or taken a test or gone to therapy or interacted with a friend, I leave those situations/interactions with the voice in my brain telling me that I suck, and I hate myself in one way or another. In the periods of my life when I was extremely depressed, I was literally unable to leave my bed for months in part because the self-hatred felt so strong, and I believed all of the negative things I thought about myself. I also overanalyze every single behavior / interaction / characteristic about myself until I have turned it into something terrible."*

Answer 2: "*My entire identity was trapped within my self-loathing, and it probably contributed to the majority of my symptoms. How does a person function normally when they don't believe they deserve to exist? Obviously, I became horrifically depressed, and my entire world came crashing down along with my mood. It's a domino effect. My self-hatred caused my relationships with my friends to suffer–I needed constant validation from them that they cared because I didn't understand how anyone could care. But what teenager wants to deal with a person like that? So, I lost all of my friends. I couldn't get myself to go to school anymore, even though I was in a special charter school for health care that I absolutely loved. The only reason I graduated was because the district hired private tutors for all my classes. I dabbled in eating disorders and started cutting because of the self-loathing. My mom continued to berate me or roll her eyes. My dreams of becoming a nurse became impossible, which changed the entire trajectory of my life and continued to be a source for the self-hatred. It all became so intertwined that it's difficult, even now, to determine what has caused what. That being said, I whole-heartedly believe that the self-hatred/loathing has been one of the biggest contributing factors to the mess my life has been.*"

Answer 3: "*I think self-loathing has crippled my self-confidence, which has affected me both personally (relationships) and professionally because it has created an extreme avoidance to any sort of risk, appraisal and outside judgement which has prevented me from applying myself meaningfully in anything that I do. I am in constant fear of being judged and deemed unworthy, or garnering criticism that would support my self-hating thoughts.*"

Answer 4: "*It came out not only as thousands of negative thoughts, but it also led to self-injurious behavior. For example, I would bang my head on the corner of my windowsill as a young kid. I would specifically hit my head on the corner because it would hurt and punish me more. Also, it would bruise my head. The bruising was important to me because it showed the world how much emotional pain,*

I was in. As I got older, I realized the damage hitting my head could do to my thinking and my overall function, so when I was thirteen, I started cutting. To this day I am trying to stop that habit. Though cutting is horrible and a habit I need to stop, the thoughts about suicide are far more dangerous. I had so many attempts. There was a time in the hospital where I would be attempting suicide daily. "I deserve it, I deserve it, I deserve it." Those words echoed through my brain constantly."

Answer 5: "*The impact it had was tremendous. Life looked and felt so dull. Everything that meant so much to me did not feel like enough to stay alive for. It became so hard to function I felt like my only option was suicide. I mean it had been years and years built up of this absolute disgust toward myself. Life became too hard, and my emotions became too big, so at school I had my first attempt that almost killed me. I had had plenty of attempts starting at thirteen years old but this one was different. I landed in the emergency trauma room at the ER (Emergency room). Because I had hung myself in the school bathroom. I was left in a neck brace for weeks. This truly almost killed me."*

Answer 6: "*Self-loathing has greatly impacted my sense of self because it has caused me to feel worthless, going so far as to feel undeserving of being alive. It has impacted my ability to function through developing a debilitating eating disorder and depression, that has caused me to lose interest in many things I used to enjoy and feel extreme fatigue. Self-loathing has also caused me to internalize any and all constructive criticism as indications of fundamental flaws in my character, which has only intensified my self-loathing."*

Answer 7: "*I don't really connect with the idea of having a sense of self, but any sense of self I do have is grounded in having no worth, being deserving of bad things, and anger towards myself. I think that despite my self-loathing, my functioning externally has remained objectively high. However, it has had a significant negative impact on my enjoyment of and sense of achievement around my accomplishments in life. It feels as though nothing I do will ever by good enough for me, and I have very little in terms of a sense of ownership over my accomplishments. I often feel as though I don't deserve the accomplishments or like they were given to me out of pity because I am a pathetic person and there is no way I could have actually accomplished something on my own."*

Answer 8 (a master's level student): *"The interpersonal theory of suicide says that suicidality is related to thwarted belongingness and perceived burdensomeness. In my experience, suicidality and self-hatred are intertwined, and I believe that both concepts are also related to my self-hatred. My experience of disability is extremely relevant to how I relate to these concepts. I grew up with undiagnosed medical problems/disability that resulted in, among other things, unexplained mobility limitations, high levels of pain, and frequent illness. Practically, this looked like things such as missing school more frequently, being worse at sports, and overall having lower stamina. This was, of course, noticed by my peers. The results of the whole situation as they relate to belongingness were twofold. First, I was not able to participate in physically challenging group activities, for example games in PE class or soccer at recess, in the ways that everyone else could, which made me feel separated socially and like I was not like other kids. Second, other kids often thought I was making up my problems for attention, which resulted in even more socially ostracization."*

"My experiences with perceived burdensomeness and disability came into being later in my life than the thwarted belonginess. Retrospectively, it first became a noticeable problem when I was a teenager and peaked around the time I was 21 or 22. I didn't start seeking answers for my health problems in my mid-teens. I went to countless appointments and worked my way through many different specialties. I sometimes went for tests that were complicated and took hours. I usually scheduled all my appointments myself, and once I was old enough to drive, I took myself to all my appointments on my own as well. When a test required my dad to come with me because I wouldn't be allowed to drive after, I felt incredibly guilty."

"I felt as though I was not deserving of the time that my dad had to take out of his day to physically be there for me. I also tried to hide my physical pain from my parents, as I didn't think they deserved the psychological burden of having a sick child. So yeah, the medical stuff which compounded my already-existing self-hatred, made suicide a reasonable solution. I don't think that I would have thought about suicide without the self-hatred, because I would have had more compassion for the way in which I was suffering physically."

At its core, self-loathing occupies a lot of thought space and can declare its enduring presence at any moment.

> "Why are you lying awake, thinking that you're a terrible person?"
>
> "To keep my mind occupied when I can't sleep. Some people count sheep. I self-loathe."
>
> —Rainbow Rowell

Clearly, living day-in and day-out with enduring self-loathing has impact beyond simply having a bad day. It colors all aspects of a person's life. It's so evident that this has to be addressed because it leads to immeasurable suffering, and even when a person is in therapy, very few clinicians talk about it with their patients or even amongst themselves. Addressing and overcoming self-hatred means that people who experience it, will suffer less.

B) The Risk of Suicide

> "I have such intense self-hatred that I want to be dead. Death is the only thing that will end it."
>
> —Patient with lived experience

Research

Feeling a burden to others

When a research team (Turnell et al. 2019), developed a scale to assess self-hatred in clinical populations, the team found that high levels of self-hatred predicted suicidal ideation. Participants reported this was often because of the sense of being a burden to others and also of not having a sense of belonging. This finding is particularly relevant for people who have conditions like borderline personality disorder (BPD see Chapter 8) as they often struggle with suicidal thoughts, feel that they are a burden to others, and that they don't belong. And so, when this is compounded by self-hatred, the risk of suicide increases significantly.

Other research has suggested that suicidal thoughts and behaviors often function as a way to escape aversive and unwanted emotions. People with BPD and related conditions experience very strong emotions, to the point that the emotions can feel even more painful than the sensation of severe physical pain. Because the emotions appear to be triggered by seemingly the smallest of provocations, any feelings of self-hatred will make the entire experience excruciating. When this happens, at times, suicide seems like the perfect way to end the pain and suffering.

Often, when I initially meet people with self-hatred and I ask them how they are doing, they say "fine" and in the majority of cases, "fine" is the furthest thing from how they are feeling. But how is the outside observer to know? The person with self-hatred does not show the manic symptoms of someone with bipolar disorder, the poor self-care of someone with depression, the distractibility of someone with ADHD, the ritualistic behavior of someone with obsessive compulsive disorder or the intoxicated behavior of someone addicted to substances. How can anyone help or respond when a person says that they are doing fine and there are no outward signs someone is suffering with the unbearable pain of self-hatred.

The pain is only revealed when the person articulates it, and even when they do, many offer a counter perspective: "How is this possible, you are so loved, so intelligent, have such a great job, have friends, etc. etc." These well-meaning statements add further fuel to the self-hatred fire because the person with self-loathing thinks "exactly. So, why should I complain? I am so ungrateful."

In most cases, the suffering caused by self-hatred is not visible to others, but the experience of it is so painful, that the person will do anything to alleviate it. One patient told me: *"I had bone cancer as a child, and that was painful. But I would rather have that pain, than the pain of self-hatred. When you have bone cancer, there are medications, and also people understand that you're in pain. They see it in the bone scans and blood tests. My self-hatred pain is worse than that. There are no medications, unless I take way more than prescribed to numb myself, and there are no blood tests, or scans. It's unseen and quiet. And unbearable. And it hurts."*

Many people who can't conceptualize how suicide could ever be a solution, are mystified by this. I completely agree. SUICIDE IS NOT A SOLUTION. Nevertheless, I often ask my colleagues and the family members of my patients to consider the following thought experiment.

Think about a time that was unbearably painful for you emotionally. Maybe it was the loss of a loved one, a false accusation, divorce, the loss of a job and so on. Think about the emotional pain you suffered. Now imagine that I said to you that you will feel that pain for the rest of your life. When people consider the most emotionally painful experiences of their life, the thought of having to endure that much pain seems unimaginable and many say that if they absolutely knew that it would be that way forever, that it seems like the unending pain of some debilitating physical illness, and that then, yes, they could see how someone might consider suicide. That is how bad it can feel for people with enduring self-hatred.

Compounded by Maltreatment

Another study (Nilsson et al. 2022) divided patients into 3 groups. One group had 34 people who had psychiatric diagnoses and who also self-harmed, the second group had 31 people with psychiatric diagnoses, but who did *not* self-harm, and the third was a group of 29 people who had neither a psychiatric diagnosis, nor self-harm.

The three groups were compared using measures of self-harm, childhood maltreatment, attitudes toward themselves and attitudes toward self-harm. The researchers found the group of 34 patients who self-harmed reported more emotional abuse and more self-hatred compared to the two other groups. The emotional impact of the childhood abuse was made even worse by self-hatred. People who self-harmed had a far more positive attitude toward self-harm than those who did not self-harm. The authors concluded that self-hatred and emotional abuse in childhood could be a distinguishing characteristic of patients who self-harm and supported the hypothesis that emotional abuse leads to self-harm because of the experience of the self-hatred.

What I found particularly interesting in their conclusion was this statement: "Finally, there is still a need to improve treatments for self-hatred and we therefore urge clinicians to try to explore and develop novel approaches towards this end since self-hatred, according to this study, might be of particular importance for suffering in this population." Exactly right!

Havoc

> "Oh my life is so awful, it's just so awful to be me, you don't know what it's like waking every morning and finding the whole horror of being yourself still there."
>
> —Iris Murdoch

In the context of the scant research, we recently published a paper (Wilner et al. 2024) to shine a spotlight on self-hatred. With the experience causing havoc on a sense of self, disruptions in a relational life, an academic life, a work life as well as the sense of being a burden and not belonging, and all of which lead to the conclusion that suicide is the only solution, it is crystal clear that overcoming self-hatred and addressing it directly has to be a central focus. Living with this chronic symptom is not acceptable and whether you are tackling it on your own or in therapy, collectively we need to do all we can to help you see yourself for the potential that you are. In the next chapter, I will delve deeper into the signs and symptoms of self-hatred.

Chapter 3

Common Signs of Self-Hatred

"I won't sleep, if that's what it takes, to not wake up as myself."

—Casey Renee Kiser

Sometimes self-hatred is so pervasive that you are not thinking about it except for when things go wrong, or when you imagine things are your fault or that you are to blame for everything. Nevertheless, there are some common signs and symptoms that people with self-loathing experience. This chapter focuses on these experiences and examines them more broadly. My goal in this chapter is for you to begin to move from an automatic "I HATE MYSELF" to a more examined and introspective stance.

Before reviewing some of the more common experiences, take some time to examine your experience of self-hatred.

Questions About Your Experience

If you go to a therapist, it is likely that you will be asked questions about the quality and amount of sleep you get, the amount of energy you have, if you have suicidal thoughts, how much you are eating, if you are losing weight, if you are hearing voices, and so on. However, because enduring self-hatred has not been well-studied, and because as therapists we are not trained to ask about self-hatred, it is NOT typically addressed in standard initial mental health evaluations or therapy. It stands to reason that if you are not asked about it, that you won't talk about it and if you don't talk about it, that you will continue to struggle with it.

1. In any psychiatric assessment or evaluation, have you ever been asked about self-loathing/self-hatred? Y/N
2. How far back do you remember the feelings of self-loathing?

____

3. What does, or did, your self-loathing look like?

____

____

____

4. How would you describe it to others?

____

____

5. How intense or enduring are, or were, the feelings?

____

____

6. How do you think your self-hatred started?

____

____

____

____

7. Did something specific happen to you, or did the feelings develop over time?

____

____

8. How has self-loathing impacted your sense of self and your overall functioning/experience of life?

____

____

____

____

____

9. Did you ever think of practicing self-compassion or self-love? Y/N

a. If yes, how did you hear about self-compassion and what was your experience of the practice?

b. If no, why not?

10. Are there times or circumstances that shift your experience of self-loathing, ones that make it more or less intense? What are these?

____

____

____

____

11. If you are further along in your journey, and if you have noticed a reduction in self-loathing:

a. Did you do something specific to target it? Y/N and if so what?

____

____

____

b. If you are in therapy, and it hasn't been brought up, can you tell your therapist that you want to start tackling it? Y/N

c. What would you tell others who struggle with self-loathing about what works and what does not?

____

____

____

d. Do you ever worry that it will come back? Y/N

Breaking It Down Further

There are various signs and symptoms that can be conceptually categorized together. Your task is to reflect on these and reflect on the exercises as fully as you can.

- **All-or-nothing thinking:** Extreme versions of this would be, for example, if you make some minor mistake and then you feel that your life is ruined, that you are a failure, and that you are solely to blame.

  One of my patients, someone who had never missed an appointment, was scheduled last minute to do an extra shift at work. The issue was that the extra shift took place during our regularly scheduled meeting time. However, because she was not sure that her work valued her, being given an extra shift made her feel better about herself and seen as a part of her work team. In this context, she forgot to cancel her appointment with me. Because she had never missed, or if needing to cancel in advance, I was worried and texted her to make sure she was okay. She immediately texted back: "I am so sorry. I am such a terrible person. This is exactly why you should fire me. I am such a disappointment. I can't get anything right." Her one, completely understandable omission led her to think that if she could not get this one thing right, she could get nothing right.

  One day, another of my patients came in to session crying, telling me that everyone hated her. She was so upset. I asked her what had happened, and she told me that it was her 35th birthday and that neither of her brothers had sent her a card, and that all she had received was a very late-night text from them. "I don't think they remembered. I think that my mom told them to send me a text. They don't love me. They hate me." Later it turned out that one brother, who "never remembers anything," had in fact forgotten her birthday and he felt miserable about doing so, and her other brother HAD sent her a card, and it was in her mailbox. Her thinking that they either loved her or they hated her, is another example of black-or-white thinking, and in her case, it led her to the painful conclusion that everyone hated her.

Maybe you can identify with these examples, but there are plenty of other ways this style of thinking could play out in your internal dialogue, even without realizing it. Do you tend to see situations in extreme terms, without recognizing any middle ground? Telltale signs include using absolute language such as "always" and "never," perceiving what others may view as minor mistakes as total failures, and thinking in opposites, like seeing yourself as either a complete success or an utter failure. This mindset can lead to unrealistic expectations and emotional distress when the idea of perfection is not achieved.

EXERCISE

Is all-or-nothing thinking a part of your experience? If so, what are examples in your life?

YOUR ANSWER:

___

___

___

- **Focusing on the negative:** This is the tendency to focus on the negative of every situation.

In another session, this same patient told me that she had had a productive day at work and that her boss had told her that she was doing a great job and then what she would need to do to get a promotion. Instead of appreciating her boss's recognition, she instead focused on what her boss expected of her in order to get the promotion. She interpreted her boss's expectation as negative criticism and then focused her attention on all the things that she wasn't doing.

The problem is that only focusing on the negative paints your world in very bleak ways. If you live in a dark cave all your life, you won't see the beauty that daylight exposes. When you are sitting in a negative state and making an inventory of all the negative, write them down, AND also write down the positives of the situation. If you can't see the positives, ask a friend or colleague for help.

EXERCISE

Do you tend to focus on the negative? If so, what are some examples in your life?

YOUR ANSWER:

____

____

____

- **Emotional reasoning:** This is the experience of having a feeling and then coming to a conclusion about a situation solely based on that feeling.

  For one of my patients, being recognized on her birthday is extremely important for her. She never forgets any of her friends' or family's birthdays and goes to great efforts to recognize them. On one occasion, she had been doing extensive travel for work, and forgot to call her sister on her birthday. She felt extremely angry at herself, and the feeling of self-loathing surged. On the basis of these feelings, she concluded that she was a terrible sister. She reasoned that because she had so much self-anger and self-hatred, that she was in "fact" a terrible sister.

Emotional reasoning has the quality of equating emotion with fact. For example, you feel anxious walking into your doctor's office and think "I feel anxious, so I know that she is going to give me bad news," or "my friend didn't offer to buy me a cup of coffee, so obviously I am not that important to her." By equating reality with how you feel, you are setting yourself up for enduring suffering because people with self-hatred often experience life negatively and so the conclusions they make about situations tend to be negative.

EXERCISE

Does this resonate and what are examples in your life?

YOUR ANSWER:

____

____

____

- **Seeking approval and constant reassurance:** Although you do not feel worthy of care or love, at the same time you constantly seek approval and reassurance from others to say that you are worth something. The problem is that this approval is very short-lived, and you then you are searching for more. It can be emotionally draining to be waiting for this reassurance because of the anxiety and desperation you feel when you don't get it. Although it helps a bit for a short period of time, you tend to believe people who are critical of you rather than the ones who truly care about you.

  When I first started to practice dialectical behavior therapy (DBT), one of my patients would constantly ask me if I cared about her. In those days, I would say that I did. I realized that she would ask me more and more. I asked my DBT colleagues about this behavior and they told me that she was seeking reassurance for something that was important to her. Rather than me telling her that I did, her task was to internalize the knowledge that her recovery, her mental health, and her success was important to me without asking for reassurance. I explained this to her, and she thought that my not reassuring her meant that I hated her, but once she was able to realize and validate the hard work she was doing without needing my reassurance, she increasingly began to see her self-worth.

For most people, receiving positive feedback makes us happy. However, constantly seeking approval and reassurance is a sign that you may be dependent on validation from others to feel confident and secure. If you start to feel anxious or uncertain without external affirmation you may depend on others' opinions instead of providing these yourself, which can lead to doubting your own judgment and needing continual encouragement to feel reassured. This often happens when chronic invalidation has caused you to be uncertain about the truth of your experience. This is known as self-invalidation. If you are constantly asking: "Do you think I did the right thing?" or "Are you sure I'm good enough?" this can lead to a cycle of dependency on others for your self-worth, and many people with self-hatred feel that if they don't get answers to these questions, that the lack of answers proves that they are worthless.

EXERCISE

Do you tend to constantly seek approval or reassurance? If so, what are some examples in your life?

YOUR ANSWER:

____

____

____

- **You won't accept compliments, or you feel as if you are allergic to them:** If someone says something nice about you or one of your accomplishments, you discount what they say and think: "They have to say that" or "they are just being nice." This one is the opposite of always wanting reassurance.

  Although sometimes people say nice things just to be nice, most are honest, and you telling them that they don't actually believe what they are saying or are outright lying to you can be dismissive of the other person. One of my patients had been working hard on regulating her emotions by using newly acquired emotions-regulation skills. In a family meeting, her father recognized her hard work, and this caused her to leave the room. She admitted that she hated people complimenting her especially for something that she felt should be easy to do. It can aggravate self-hatred when the person concludes that they are being praised for something that they should be able to do. *"To me it feels like someone has praised me for being able to use a fork. I'm not a toddler,"* quipped a patient.

EXERCISE

Do you tend to reject compliments or feel "allergic" to them? Can you expand on this?

YOUR ANSWER:

____

____

____

- **Doing all you can to fit in:** Because you feel empty or different or like an outsider, you do all you can to fit in. Now it can be adaptive to try to fit in but sometimes you do things that cross your values, or you really aren't interested in, just to fit in. You worry excessively that if you don't do these things that people won't like you, think that you are weird or annoying, and then won't want to spend time with you, which unfortunately reinforces the idea that you are worthless.

A patient of mine was the only male in a DBT skills training group. He had a very poor sense of himself and one of his behaviors was to do what others did as a way to fit in. He enjoyed sports and especially talking about the Boston Celtics and would often use sports related examples when talking about skills in group. "The Celtics lost the other night, but rather than dwelling on the loss, I radically accepted that they had and was able to distract by listening to a podcast," he explained. The rest of the group was not interested in sports and instead was watching a Netflix show on how the Dallas Cowboys cheerleaders are selected. He desperately wanted to fit in, and decided to start watching the show even though it never interested him. The rest of the group was then more welcoming; however, he never did tell them that the only reason he was watching it was to fit in, and he felt as disconnected as ever. The pattern here is of valuing external opinion and disregarding internal preferences. But if you think about it, there are eight billion other people on the planet, each with external opinions, and only you with your specific likes. Of course, there may be other people with shared interests, but if you never share your likes and wants, how will you ever find them? It can be lonely, when you don't have common interests to share, but it is often even lonelier to pretend to be interested in things that you aren't.

EXERCISE

Do you spend a lot of time trying to fit in by copying others' behaviors and fashions, even when they don't completely match who you are? Say more about this:

YOUR ANSWER:

____

____

____

- **Taking any sort of feedback as criticism or a personal attack:** You take recommendations, suggestions, and feedback as a personal attack. What's worse is that this not only happens in the moment, but long after the event took place.

  On one occasion, I was marveling at a patient's writing. It was so good, that I felt that she should consider publishing it. As I handed it back to her, I saw a minor typo. She wrote "where" instead of "were." I congratulated her on her writing. Also, knowing that she would feel judged if someone else had found it, I pointed out the minor error. Later she texted me that my observation was all that she could think about, that I thought that she was stupid and unable to spell, and that my criticism pointed out just how flawed she was.

  She told me that she felt judged, and then hurt, and then angry with me. She interpreted my pointing it out as underscoring her ineptitude. The intent of the feedback was lost. "Intentions don't matter," she told me.

EXERCISE

Do you tend to see feedback, even constructive feedback, as negative or a personal attack? Think about this for yourself. Think of a time when someone gave you feedback that felt critical. What was your emotional response? Do you find it difficult to accept any advice? What are some examples in your life?

YOUR ANSWER:

____

____

____

____

____

- **Bringing others down:** Either because of envy, jealousy, or feeling bad about yourself, you bring others down with the intention of making the other person feel bad, and in so doing feeling better about yourself. When this particular symptom happens, it is done with intention.

  One patient gave me an example of this. A friend of hers had been invited to a party that she had not been invited to. Her friend was telling her all about it, and she noticed an increasing amount of envy. My patient told me that she could not stand how happy her friend was, because with each account of the party, she felt more and more worthless. "I am so glad I got invited," said her friend. Envy and jealousy boiling over, my patient said: "That's great. It probably doesn't happen so often given how fat you are." Her friend left the house crying and at first, my patient felt great that someone was suffering as much as she was, but later felt very guilty and called her friend to apologize. Another patient told me that he wanted me to know how much he suffered and that he could not think of what else to do than to devalue me. "You think that you're a great psychiatrist, but you're not. I wish my other psychiatrist was still working so that I could have a real psychiatrist." I suggested that he could look for someone else, and he retorted, "You see what I mean, now you want to abandon me just like so many have done. You have no idea how painful that statement was." His behavior of devaluation significantly adversely impacted our relationship. He felt terrible that he had been so mean. "You see. Look at the terrible things I say. I am a terrible, despicable person and don't deserve to live." He was a young man who had been devalued his whole life, always compared to the successes of his older siblings, and devaluation was the only thing that he knew to do to elicit pain in others. After a few months of learning about self-validation, his verbal attacks diminished, and he successfully completed therapy.

EXERCISE

Do you have a tendency to want others to feel as bad as you are feeling and then do behaviors that diminish them? What are some examples?

YOUR ANSWER:

____

____

____

- Fearing healthy connections: You push away friends or lovers, those who could be healthy people in your life, fearing that you will get too close to them and that they will discover what an awful person you are and then leave you. On the other hand, you accept unacceptable behavior from abusive people feeling that you deserve the abuse, or that the abusive relationship is the best one you can get or expect.

  Some months after a patient had gone through a painful breakup, she told me that she had met a new person at work. The person was kind and considerate and seemed to listen. The closer she got to the work colleague, the more she feared that the colleague would discover, like her former partner had, "what a terrible person I am," and in this context, abruptly quit her job as she feared she was getting too close to the colleague and that someone like her did not deserve a healthy relationship.

EXERCISE

Are you worried that by getting close to anyone, they will discover what an "awful" person you are? If so, what are some examples?

YOUR ANSWER:

____

____

____

- **Being afraid of having, or refusing to have, big dreams and goals:** This can occur when you feel so bad about yourself that you don't believe that anything will ever work out, or that if you go for something big, that you will inevitably fail. Then any success that you do achieve, you attribute to luck rather than to your hard work.

  One patient told me: "I never thought about life beyond my 18th birthday. I didn't think I'd be alive. I thought that I was such a burden that removing myself from the world would be the kindest thing I could do. Now that I care about myself, life is weird. I mean if you have never had dreams, how do you start having them now?"

  "How do you feel about that?" I asked.

  "I am so glad that I am still here to find out!" they responded.

EXERCISE

Do you struggle with, or avoid, dreaming big or setting up life goals? How does this manifest in your life?

YOUR ANSWER:

____

____

____

- **Being overly self-critical:** If you make a mistake, you have a very hard time being kind to yourself, and instead tend to take full blame for what happened, or attribute negative outcomes to negative self-characteristics, without recognizing any positivity in yourself. You refuse to consider other possible outside factors.

  I was asked to consult with a patient on the inpatient unit. He had been admitted after a suicide attempt. He had been part of a team submitting a proposal to their company, and he relied on another team member to provide the data they needed for their proposal. The data was incorrect, and he only discovered this at the presentation. He felt solely responsible for the failure, felt that it reflected his incompetence, and could not hear the feedback that the proposal had merit, and that the error should be corrected and re-presented. Instead, he felt that his life was over and that he could do nothing right.

EXERCISE

Do you have a tendency to beat yourself up whenever you make a mistake? No matter how small a mistake it is? Or even if it is a perceived mistake? If so, what are some examples?

YOUR ANSWER:

____

____

____

There are other signs and symptoms that you might experience, and if you have some that are different from the previous example, write them down here:

____

____

Chain Analysis: A Tool for Recognizing the Factors That Cause Problematic Behavior

Now that you've identified occasions when self-hate has become all encompassing, you're likely to recognize that these situations are ones that are stressful. Here is a practice that can help you recognize the vulnerability factors, thoughts, behaviors, and interactions that show up early in the sequence of events that lead to the magnification of self-hatred.

DBT is a type of therapy that teaches skills to help people manage strong emotions, more effectively tolerate difficult moments, reduce destructive behaviors, and improve relationships. (I'll review DBT more comprehensively later in the book.) One of the tools used in DBT is known as a chain analysis to understand behavior. It tracks and identifies the moment-to-moment sequence of events, including the thoughts, feelings, and behaviors that lead to problematic behaviors, using an ABC model. ABC is an acronym that stands for the Antecedents (things that come before the behavior), the actual Behavior, and the Consequences (the things that come after the behavior). It is an active process where a therapist and their patient look for the "active ingredients" for a problem behavior.

For example, let's say that a person was feeling sad, very lonely, and unwanted and then went out to a bar one night and impulsively hooked up with the first person that showed them any interest. They just wanted to feel less alone, and the loneliness was so painful that they did not consider the potential dangers of the hookup. The therapist and patient decide to analyze the hookup behavior and use the ABC model of chain analysis to understand the behavior in a more complete way.

a. **A**ntecedents are the elements that happen *before* the problematic behavior. These can include the location (bar), people (stranger), time of day (night), and internal circumstances (e.g., emotions [sad], thoughts [I am lonely]) that occur before the behavior.

b. **B**ehavior is the actual problematic behavior: The hookup.

c. **C**onsequences are the elements of experience that happen as a result of the behavior, both short-term and long-term, intended and unintended. For instance, there may be some instant relief of the loneliness as a short-term consequence, but then some self-disgust as a longer-term consequence. Perhaps, the person experiences an unintended consequence such as an infection, or maybe there is an intended consequence, feeling that they wanted to feel punished, and felt so after the hookup.

What does ABC have to do with self-loathing? For people with chronic self-hatred, sometimes the experience flares up because of some interaction with another, and then this leads to problematic behavior. For instance, say you feel criticized at work and then notice a flare-up of self-hatred and then drink heavily to numb the feeling. In this case, self-hatred would be an antecedent to the behavior. Alternatively, say you go out with friends, and they are all speaking badly about another friend in the group, one who is not there. You join in with them, trashing the absent friend. The next day, you think about the behavior of speaking poorly about your friend, know that having done so crosses your values, and then notice a spike in self-hatred. In this case, self-hatred comes *after* the behavior and is a consequence of the behavior.

Of course, self-hatred can be both an antecedent and consequence. Understanding when in a sequence of events self-hatred intensifies can help you consider situations that might make you more vulnerable to the experience and then deal with them when you are feeling less emotional so self-hatred doesn't intensify.

Let's end this chapter where we started it: Sometimes self-hatred is so pervasive that you are not thinking about it except for when things go wrong, or when you imagine things are your fault or that you are to blame for everything. Nevertheless, there are some common signs and symptoms that people with self-loathing experience. By becoming aware of these signs and symptoms, you can start to recognize patterns and triggers in your own behavior. This awareness is the first step toward breaking the cycle of self-hate and then beginning to think and behave in ways that are more consistent with self-care and eventually self-compassion.

In the next chapter you'll hear the voices of people who live with self-loathing as a core part of their self and their daily experience.

Chapter 4

The Lived Experience

"As incompetent in life as in death, I loathe myself, and in this loathing, I dream of another life, another death. And for having sought to be a sage such as never was, I am only a madman among the mad. . . ."

—Emil Cioran, *A Short History of Decay*

At the core of self-hatred is the thought: "I hate myself." I want to underscore that it is, after all, a thought. Why is defining it as a thought important? A thought is a representation of something. Think about a table. In your mind you have created a likeness or concept that stands in for something that has certain characteristics such as a piece of furniture with a flat top supported by four legs. I could, of course, show you tables with one central support, one with three legs or one with more than four legs. The point is that the thought "table" is a representation separate from the actual object. Of course, you could become far more descriptive: "I am thinking of a round table, made of cherry wood, with four tapered legs, that is three feet wide."

In terms of communication to yourself and other people, you can see that there is a clear difference between saying "I am thinking about a table" and the descriptive version. The more descriptive you are, the more information you are imparting, whether to yourself or others.

How would you experience self-hatred if you had to break down the thought in a descriptive way including all its elements so that you could explain it to others?

Self-loathing declares itself through consistent and repetitive negative thoughts that are closely tied to excessive self-criticism, self-blame, and self-disgust. While self-criticism can be a healthy assessment of one's behavior, it can start to overshadow and then overwhelm other thought patterns, in particular when you're in the throes of a self-deprecating cycle. People who live with self-hatred know its impact on thoughts, emotions, behaviors, relationships, and so many other aspects of life.

In this chapter, at the end of each exercise, I have added the action item "INSIGHT." Your task is to see if you can reflect on the accuracy of your experience and see if there is another, wiser conclusion.

Impact on Thoughts

When I asked about the experience and the persistence of the thoughts, one patient told me: *"They are constant. They filled my brain to the brim with self-deprecating thoughts and there was no escape. The language of self-loathing became who I was. Saying positive things to myself felt uncanny. I found comfort in negative thinking habits. Saying I was the worst or that I hate myself, in a way, felt better than saying I was a good person, or even a fine person. I would, at times, try to challenge them as I got older, but I would just let up. They became me. How could I change the language I learned so young? It was not going to be easy. Especially since I thought it was impossible. I could not imagine a life without it. I was not just telling myself these things; people were also telling me that I was a bad person."*

EXERCISE

Consider the ways that self-hatred has impacted how you think. What are the specific thoughts related to self-hatred and other aspects of your life?

YOUR ANSWER:

____

____

____

____

____

INSIGHT: Now that you have answered this question, is there a way to consider the automatic ways in which your self-hatred thoughts arise? What questions do you have about how they have developed over time? Spend a few minutes reflecting on your experience of the question and your answer and see if there are other ways of considering your experience.

Thoughts Lead to Emotions Lead to Behaviors

Some years ago, a patient came for DBT treatment, and her therapist asked me to talk to her about her self-hatred. I asked the patient to tell me about her experience and whether she was willing to challenge the idea that self-hatred was a fixed part of who she was. She said she wanted to think about it for a day. So many of the stories I hear from patients have the familiar theme of believing that changing core self-hatred is not possible. Here's what she told me the next day:

> *"You asked me to consider the mere possibility that I could be wrong about my belief that self-hatred is me. That the dialog that I have so tirelessly maintained could be flawed. Flawed in both reasoning and within the premise itself. You asked me to look at the little girl that I used to be. I did. I imagined her looking in the mirror and I drowned in the longing to cut her stomach off with scissors. Would I give her those scissors today? No, of course not. But today, do I drown in the same desperate desire? Yes, and if it were a rational possibility, I would act on it as well.*
>
> *How is it that we are always changing yet the dialog I created so long ago seems to remain constant? How is it possible that the little girl that I once was already carried the weight of unavoidable shame from a guilt that had yet to be discovered?*
>
> *No harm no foul right? Apparently not. Where was the harm? Was it the mere fact of my existence? But looking at that little girl, how could I say that? I don't hate her today so why did I hate her*

then? However, I deeply hate myself now. In 20 years when I look back at pictures of myself now will I feel the same as I do looking at 5-year-old me? If in 20 years I look back and ask myself, 'how could you hate that young woman?' then what the fuck is the point and why am I so stuck in this dialog that is slowly seeming less logical?

My dialog of self-hatred was unknowingly created and unwillingly strengthened through years of invalidation, inflicted pain, and outright assault. The issue is that no matter how this dialog came to be, I have knowingly been maintaining it with every fiber within myself. Every thought, followed by many feelings, and far too many behaviors have acted as evidence to help the loathing grow.

Hate is a strong word. But it doesn't come close to describing how I have grown to feel about myself. The dialog that was created, maintained, and strengthened is more harmful than anything I have ever known. The pain is insufferable.

Yet here I am. I still hate myself. And I hate myself so much that it's hard for me to believe that I shouldn't hate myself. But you did ask me to consider that maybe, just maybe, my dialog is wrong.

So here I am … considering it."

The impact of thoughts is powerful. Thoughts can lead to adaptive and pro-compassion behaviors; however, for people with self-hatred, it is the negative thoughts about themselves that lead to self-hatred. A negative thought is any thought that leaves you feeling upset or worse about yourself. People who have experienced abuse, rejection, or invalidation are much more likely to have negative thoughts, and these thoughts can trigger powerful and often painful emotions including anxiety, anger, sadness, guilt, shame, or fear. In order to deal with these unwanted emotions, some turn to destructive behaviors such as drugs, alcohol, self-injury, avoidance, and many others. Although these behaviors can reduce intensity of the emotions in the short run, they often cause people to feel worse in the long run, which then causes the person to feel even worse about themselves, which can entrench the idea that they are flawed and terrible people and eventually lead to self-hatred. And so, if you start paying attention to the cycle that starts with negative thoughts, and label it as a cycle, you are taking a first step in breaking from a self-destructive cycle, and this in turn is an act of kindness to yourself.

EXERCISE

Do your thoughts lead to strong emotions? Do these in turn lead to destructive behaviors? What are some examples?

YOUR ANSWER:

____

____

____

____

____

INSIGHT: Now that you have answered this question, is there a way to see the connection between your thoughts of self-hatred, the ensuing emotions, and the resultant behavior any differently? Spend a few minutes reflecting on your answer to the question and see if destructive behavior makes sense given the evolution of your self-hatred.

Impact on Relationships

In Chapter 3, we explored the idea that people with self-hate often come to the conclusion that they are not worthy of a positive relationship. This can create a cognitive dissonance: If you don't like yourself and yet others tell you that you are likeable, the mental discomfort that arises from holding two conflicting beliefs can be confusing at best, and very painful at worst, if you believe that they are lying. The certainty that you are unlikeable clashes against the insistence of others telling you that you are likeable.

What are you to conclude if someone tells you that they like you? I have posed this question to various people who experience self-hatred, and these are the typical answers:

- **a.** "They are lying."
- **b.** "Maybe they are not lying, but they don't see the real me. If they did, they would not like me."
- **c.** "They are saying they like me to be nice."
- **d.** "They have to say it because they are my family/friends."
- **e.** "They don't want to hurt my feelings by telling me the truth."
- **f.** "If I am truly likeable and everyone can see it but me, it shows that I am crazy and who likes crazy people?"

"So, are your parents or friends lying to you when then say that they genuinely like you?" I asked a patient.

"Maybe they are lying, but I don't think that it is exactly that. They just see what they see. If they knew how terrible I am, they would hate me as much as I hate myself. I just don't trust the answer because either, yes, they are lying, or they are so clueless about me that they have terrible judgment," she said.

"So, trust is relevant? How has self-loathing impacted your ability to trust others?" I asked.

"I think that because I think so poorly of myself, I assume everyone else feels the same. With that assumption in the forefront of my mind when meeting potential friends, I am less likely to trust them because I think they don't like me, or if they say they do, that they have poor judgment, so how can I trust them?" she answered.

"You have told me that there are people in the world that you would consider to be truly evil given what they have done. You are also telling me that if people really knew you, that they would see just how awful a person you are. All I hear from your parents and your friends is how wonderful you are, how caring you are, how thoughtful you are. You tell me they don't

know you. When are you doing all the terrible things that make you terrible? Do you sneak out in the middle of the night when no one can see you and do hateful things and then come back home and be the nice person you are? With all the awful people in the world, the serial killers, the corrupt conmen, the abusive coaches, and so on, their deeds are part of the public record and can be attested to by others. You still haven't told me the terrible things you have done that make you such a terrible person that you and others should hate you for," I insisted.

She thought for a while: "I think that it is different. I will give you that I am not terrible, and that again, maybe what I need to do is change the words that I use to describe how I feel and how I think."

I can't overstate the importance of understanding the impact of negative thinking. These negative self-representations, created by negative early experiences and perpetuated by pervasive and enduring devaluing interactions, become so deeply instilled that it is unlikely that you have either revised or even revisited how they became what you believe.

But here's my observation: When I meet the patients I work with, I like them! And when I speak to their support network, friends, family, and romantic partners, they like them, too. Of course, any one of us can be annoying or disagreeable at times, but the idea that a person is worthy of hate is rarely shared by others. Others often see and appreciate the positive qualities and potential in people who do not see it in themselves. People around them share different truths and hold positive points of view, seeing their strengths, worth, and value. These contrasting perspectives highlight that the negative self-perceptions are not definitive or absolute truths but rather the understandable, yet false, conclusions of past harm. Considering that positive feedback and perspectives from the people who care about you might be true is one of the important steps to helping erode the negativity of the past.

EXERCISE

Consider the ways that self-hatred has impacted how you see yourself in relationships. Do you insist that others cannot like you? That you are a burden to them? How do you discount the positive ways in which others see you?

YOUR ANSWER:

____

____

____

____

____

INSIGHT: Now that you have answered this question, is there a way that you can begin to imagine that you might actually be someone of worth to people who do care about you? Is it possible to recognize that maybe there are moments when you are not the best or most likeable version of yourself, and yet see that no one else is ever perfect? And in the way that you accept the best and lesser versions of others, that others might see you in this way, too. Spend a few minutes reflecting on your answer and see if you can hold in mind this idea.

Tolerating Abusive Relationships

Another experience common to people with core self-hatred is that of tolerating abusive relationships. Self-hate typically co-exists with low self-worth, and many people with low self-worth feel that they deserve any poor treatment from others. In some circumstances, people who have been abused or neglected find that abuse and neglect from new people is familiar and seems to reinforce the idea that they deserve the treatment, or alternatively that they don't deserve better. These individuals may find abusive relationships familiar and more comfortable so they will unconsciously seek out relationships that mirror their early experiences. So, they will tolerate abusive behavior from others and settle for abusive partners, thinking they do not deserve better. As I highlighted in Chapter 3 in the behaviors typical of those with self-hate, patients often seek external validation. In abusive relationships, the abuser may initially provide affection and attention, which can be mistaken for validation. However, as the abuse progresses, the person with self-hatred may continue to seek approval from the abuser, believing that any relationship is better than none at all, but with the consequence of perpetuating the cycle of self-hatred.

> *"It took me 4 years to leave my abusive relationship. It wasn't physical abuse although to be honest I sometimes wish it had been, so that others could have seen the bruises. It was mostly emotional. When I wasn't enough and I couldn't satisfy him, he would come home late from work and tell me that he had been at a bar with his friends. He would tell me about these girls who were hitting on him, and then I would do whatever he wanted to keep him. The girls where always thinner than me, prettier than me, smarter than me, less exhausted than me, more ambitious than me, more sexual than me. I hated myself even more and I could not stand how he made me feel, but I could not leave him. I became so dependent on him, and when I reached out to my family, he told me that I needed to grow up and rely on him. I was increasingly isolated. He said terrible things about my friends and colleagues, and this just underscored how useless I was. A useless person with useless friends, useless work and useless colleagues. But one morning I was sitting in my kitchen and saw a woman walking by my house, holding her partner's hand and they were laughing. And I thought to myself, 'That's what I want, and if I can't have that, I don't want the misery of my life.' I called out of work, packed my bags, and went to my parents and they hugged me and cried, and I thought that if they could love such a miserable person, then maybe I could learn to as well, and that is when I looked for a therapist."*

People who hate themselves have low self-esteem, and in this context are ultra-sensitive to any indication that someone else might consider them unworthy, unlovable, or incapable. This can then lead to one of two relational difficulties. The first is doing the wrong thing for you in order to make the other person happy. This can include tolerating abusive and hurtful behavior from the other person, which in turn can leave you thinking that you deserve the abuse and reinforces your self-hatred. The second is that rather than looking for compassionate and kind people, you might look for abusive people, feeling that they are the people you deserve in your life and that they are the only ones who would be interested in you.

EXERCISE

Consider your relationships. Does your self-hatred impact the behavior you accept and tolerate from others? Do you tend to choose abusive people, feeling that kind people would never be interested in you? Write down the impact of your self-hatred on the behavior you tolerate from others and the types of people you tend to choose.

YOUR ANSWER:

____

____

____

____

____

____

____

INSIGHT: Pay attention to the behavior you tolerate from others; you are teaching them how to treat you. Reflect on how the kind people in your life treat you and how those who are not so kind treat you. Are you effectively teaching them that it is okay to act toward you in the way that they do? Sit with this thought for a few minutes and see what new ideas arise.

Impact on Hope

I asked a patient to think about a life without self-hatred. She seemed confused by this question, and sat back then said: *"Does self-hatred ever go away? I have no clue. Does everyone deal with self-hatred? Is this something that's only tied to mental illness? There was a period in my life where I probably would have answered that I don't struggle with self-hatred. Actually, a very recent period in time! Even your asking me last week to think that it can change had me thinking "Why are we wasting time on this? I purposely sloughed off the idea because that doesn't apply to me." But then, the very second anything with my trauma is brought up, I'm suddenly painfully aware of how much I hate myself. I feel all the loathing and all the disgust that I ever had, but I have lived with it for so long that many times, I don't even really realize that it is still there. So, can it or has it ever gone away? Doubtful. Avoidance is pretty crucial. I'm just fine, IF ... Always the if."*

This patient admitted that self-loathing was causing her so much pain, particularly in the context of trauma memories, that she reluctantly, and yet willingly, agreed to consider and tackle the following:

1. That she could be deserving of love and even love herself.
2. To tackle her trauma in trauma therapy and to consider that she was not "deserving" of the trauma.
3. That the idea that she deserved to be punished for being a "bad person" was a thinking error based on years of invalidation and trauma.
4. That there would be no insistence that she practice self-compassion at any point; however, that she had to consider that the ways she thought about herself were not a choice, but the reflection of her brain biology, development, and early experiences.

Fast forward to today: She is a mom, a wife, and a healer in the medical profession, something she never imagined would ever have been possible given her self-hatred, her feeling of undeservedness, and the idea that she would never have lived long enough to see her life change because she believed it was impossible.

Self-hate will impact your sense of hope, and hopelessness will reinforce feelings of unworthiness and despair. However, as shown in this patient's example, there *is* a way forward. Through focused therapy, self-reflection, and encouragement from supportive relationships, you can begin to challenge and change your deeply ingrained negative and false beliefs. Once you start doing this, hope will rekindle. And, as with anything important worth doing, be patient with yourself. In this way, slowly, slowly the erosion of self-hatred continues.

EXERCISE

Consider how self-hatred has impacted your sense of hope and aspirations for the future. Write down the impact of your self-hatred on hope.

YOUR ANSWER:

____

____

____

____

____

INSIGHT: Even if at the moment you don't see self-hatred changing, how do you imagine your sense of hope and dreams of the future would change if you could overcome self-hatred? Reflect on this for a few minutes, and dare to consider the possibility.

Impact on an Overall Sense of Self

Clearly self-hatred has a significant impact on many aspects of a person's life. Putting it all together, here is one patient's reflection: *"For me, I don't trust people. I am unable to accept/believe compliments, it's me not believing that I'm good at anything/have any skills, it's me constantly second guessing myself, feeling constant self-doubt, blame, and disgust. When I really think about it, and hating myself so much feels like nothing I do is good enough, that I'm not capable of anything. It could be different for other people, but for me it manifested into an eating disorder and social anxiety, so yeah it really has done me a lot of damage."*

How can self-loathing not impact your sense of self? How is it possible to think that you are deserving of so many things if you feel that you are deserving of none? How can you aspire to greater dreams if you feel unworthy of attaining them? How can you imagine healthy relationships if you feel that you deserve abuse and punishment? You see, self-loathing is a terrible poison, one that pulls you away from your true self.

EXERCISE

Consider the ways that self-loathing has impacted your overall sense of who you are as a person. It's possible that you have already answered this question in the above exercises, however is there any way that is particular to you that hasn't been addressed?

YOUR ANSWER:

____

____

____

____

____

The impact can be so all consuming that it infuses every aspect of life. Here is what a young woman with an eating disorder told me: *"Self-loathing is a combination of self-criticism, self-blame, and self-disgust with chronically low self-esteem and self-worth. I feel like such a horrible, cruel person whose existence causes harm to others that I often feel like nobody wants me around and that I don't deserve to be alive. It is an all-encompassing kind of self-hatred that's uniquely directed at me; I don't experience hatred toward others in a manner even remotely close to that I experience toward myself.*"

Again and again, these narratives underscore how important it is that self-hatred be addressed and tackled directly. For some, it was the self-directed challenging of long-held beliefs, and for others the courage to bring it up in therapy. There is a path forward.

In the next chapter we are going to dive even deeper into the experience of self-hatred and consider the essential nature of self-hatred by asking, "What is the self that I am hating?"

Chapter 5

What Is the Self That You Are Hating?

This chapter is different from the others, but it is meant to provide a different lens to look through to challenge some of the long-held beliefs that are causing your pain and suffering. The stories meander and ramble a bit as I get to the point.

This is part of who I am. People who have known me for a long time tell me that when I am asked a question that requires a straightforward answer, rather than answering the question, I tend to tell a story. The reason that stories work is that they tend to illustrate points in ways that straightforward answers might not; and then, in waiting for an answer, there is an opportunity to reflect. One colleague who knows me well rolls her eyes, smiles, and says, "Oh, boy, here we go," whenever a trainee asks a question. Important questions have often been answered before, and many of these in stories. I like telling stories, and I know that they are not for everyone. I do this everywhere in life.

My son and I were watching a political debate when he asked me why it was that people seeing the very same set of facts could come to such different conclusions.

"Let me tell you a story," I said, while he rolled his eyes, "it's an old Zen short known as 'The Couple on the Donkey' and it goes like this:

> A man and his wife went into town each day, riding on their donkey.
>
> On the first day, both the wife and her husband rode on the donkey's back. When they reached the town, some of the people yelled at them. 'What is wrong with you people, putting all your weight on that poor donkey?'

The next day, having heard the criticism, the husband rode on the donkey's back and his wife walked steadily behind them. Some other people shouted, 'What kind of a man are you, forcing your wife to walk while you ride comfortably?'

And so, on the third day, they switched, and this time the wife was on the donkey's back, while the man walked behind. Again, some townspeople shouted: 'What a thoughtless man you are, leaving your wife unprotected while she rides alone.'

On the fourth day, both wife and husband walked next to the donkey. Again, some people were critical: 'What a foolish couple! Why walk if you could ride the donkey? Why even have a donkey at all?'

People can see the same set of data, the same situation, and come to different conclusions. And at times, even the person who see things one way, can see the same situation a different way the next day," I told my son.

Of course, there are so many points of view. Accommodating the ones from the people who care about you make sense, but what if you have spent a lifetime listening to the explanations of those who have hurt you, and then given those explanations the same value as all others? Discerning between helpful and aspirational perspectives, from those that do you more harm, is key to knowing what to hold on to and what to discard, and further to knowing which people to connect with and who to stay away from.

I tell stories whether I am discussing political debates with my son, or answering questions about therapy, or I am formally teaching.

Meandering

I teach dialectical behavior therapy skills to a group of parents every Monday morning with a wonderful friend, colleague, and co-teacher. Someone once asked in the group: "What is the root cause of my child's behavior?" I started by saying that in order to find the root cause of anything, we have to ask how the root cause itself arose. If a tree falls on a house during a storm, had the house not been close to the tree, or had the tree not been planted near the house, the damage would not have occurred. Why was the house built in the first place and why was the tree planted where it was?

If we imagine that a child was maltreated by its parents, we then might say that the maltreatment was the root cause of the child's psychopathology. But why did the parents maltreat their child? Was it because of how they had been raised, by parents who treated them in that way? Well then, how is it that the grandparents treated the child's parents poorly? Was it because they had adverse conditions themselves? If we go far back enough in time, had we not evolved from whatever came before us, and had life not existed on the planet, and had God or the Big Bang not created the universe, the child would not have been maltreated.

The point is that everything is caused by something, and all causes have causes. And so, rather than look for the root cause of something, it is more effective and useful to acknowledge that at times, very hurtful things have happened to all of us. We cannot go back to prevent it or change the outcome, but in this moment, right now, we can decide to not be defined by our past. Instead, we can choose to do things that line up with our values and aspirations, especially if what we are currently doing is not getting us closer to becoming the person we want to be.

I meandered for sure, to make a point, although once I finished sharing this perspective, my colleague said: "What he is saying, is that everything is caused. And that while our past has shaped us, it doesn't dictate our future entirely. We can still create meaningful and fulfilling paths forward."

What Do Stories Have to Do with the Self?

When it comes to the question of self-hatred, the topic is so enormous and so consequential that it demands more than surface-level thinking; so, let's dive right in. If you are someone who experiences profound and enduring self-loathing, see if you can be more accurate or precise in defining what you are talking about. If you say, "I hate myself," what exactly do you mean? What is this self that you are hating?

EXERCISE

Define exactly what you mean by your "self." How would you define this concept of the self?

Are you being literal in terms of all your body tissues and organs?

Do you mean your upbringing and life experiences?

Do you mean your thoughts and emotions?

The reason I want you to be very clear about this is that there are some things that you can change and others that you cannot.

For instance, you may say that you literally hate every aspect of who you are. Your kidneys, liver, heart, skin, height, eye color, and so on. Even though I ask my patients to be clear as to what they mean, I have not had a person tell me that self-hatred includes all their organs, their bone marrow, their calcium, and so on. The self is made up of many non-self elements. It is true that some feel that they are too tall, overweight, or that they have some other physical aspect that they don't like, but no one has told me that they want to discard their spleen or their esophagus in the context of things that they don't like about themselves.

So, if it is not the literal self that you are hating, when we drill down on the question of self-hatred, the answers tend to have to do more with the self reflected in unwanted thoughts and unbearable emotions that is hated. In a way, that is the good news, because thoughts and emotions are experiences that we can modify, regulate, and even change completely.

Many Years Ago

When the thought of addressing self-hatred was still in its infancy, I once asked a patient to entertain the following thought experiment: "Imagine an accident that left you without legs, would you still hate yourself?"

"Yes," she answered.

"Okay, now you are an incredibly unlucky person, and you are now in another accident, and lose your arms, still hate yourself?"

"Yes," she responded.

"You have a third accident, and you are left without all your vital organs. You are on a lung machine, heart machine, liver machine, kidney machine, and you just have your head. Still hate yourself?"

"Yup. I still do."

"But we have removed 90% of you, so what is the self you are hating?"

"It's not so much my body," she admitted. "Although I have some body dysmorphia, so sometimes I hate my body, but mostly it's my thoughts," she reflected.

"So, if we could remove your thoughts, would you still hate yourself?" I persisted.

"I hadn't thought about that. Can you do that? Aren't you your thoughts?"

"The Roman emperor Marcus Aurelius said: 'The soul becomes dyed with the color of its thoughts.' You aren't your thoughts, but certainly if your thoughts are dark and self-hateful, your being will be colored by that. But thoughts aren't fixed no matter how much you believe they are.

"Final question on this, if we replaced all your lost limbs and organs with artificial limbs and organs and the only thing that was left was your thoughts, memories, and emotions, would you still hate yourself?"

"Wow that is weird, but yes."

These are deep and complex questions that touch on the nature of identity, self-perception, and the relationship between our physical and mental self. Your identity includes your thoughts, feelings, beliefs, experiences, and how you relate to others. You might believe that your body is a vessel that changes over time, and that your core self – your consciousness, values, and inner life – remains. But this is not the case. Everything changes. When you experience self-hate, it is crucial to explore where these feelings and perceptions originated and then to challenge their validity. Whether by addressing it in therapy or by doing the exercises in this book, you continue to dismantle an idea that has caused you so much pain, and by dismantling it, you render it impotent.

Fighting Against Yourself

Now here is a very important concept, just so that you know what you are up against, especially if you are feeling suicidal and all you want to do is to kill the self, because you believe that suicide is the answer, and by the way, if I wasn't clear before, SUICIDE IS NOT THE ANSWER!

So, think about this: Some circuits in your brain talk to you about suicide. The voices are loud, so you listen to them. But what is the rest of your body doing?

Your lungs are breathing in live-giving oxygen and breathing out dangerous carbon dioxide.

Your heart is pumping oxygenated blood to every organ in your body, and then pumping blood that is low in oxygen back to your lungs in order to get more oxygen.

Your liver is filtering out toxic substances and unhealthy metabolites that arrive from the digestive system.

Your kidneys are removing waste products from your body.

Your bone marrow is producing the red blood cells that carry oxygen, the white blood cells that prevent or fight infection, and the platelets that control bleeding.

Your mitochondria are generating most of the chemical energy that is needed to power each of your cells' biochemical reactions.

And there are so many other parts of you that are doing all they can to keep you alive!

So, there is some irony that while a part of your brain is thinking that death is the answer, the rest of your body is acting to prevent that, and in doing all the healthy essential processes, is effectively saying: "That is not going to happen."

EVEN MORE OF A DIGRESSION: You can skip this section, and read the final paragraph, unless you are interested!

> "When people hate or blame you, or say hurtful things about you, look deeply into their hearts and see what kind of people they are. You'll see how unnecessary it is to want their

admiration. Even still, you must think kindly of them. They are your neighbors. The gods help them as they do you, by dreams and oracles, to win their hearts' desires."

—Marcus Aurelius

Who would have imagined that in a book on self-loathing you would be reading about Roman emperors and Greek philosophers. Marcus Aurelius was a stoic and a Roman emperor. At around the same time as Aurelius was sharing his stoic philosophy, the Greek philosopher Plutarch proposed the following thought experiment to his students. It is known as the Ship of Theseus. It goes like this:

Plutarch asked whether a ship that had been restored by replacing every single wooden part remained the same ship.

Let's just keep digging into this question. You own a boat. Imagine that you are worried about the wood on the boat, so you remove a plank of wood every few days and replace it with a new one. After you replace the first plank of wood, is it the same boat? Say that there are 100 planks of wood, and one by one you have replaced each every few days. Is it still the same boat? What if you replaced a plank every year? Does the speed of change and number of planks changed determine whether it is the same boat?

Now, a friend of yours, a carpenter, comes by and sees all the discarded planks of wood and she says: "Wow, this is great wood, why did you throw it out? It has weathered beautifully! I could build you a boat." Plank by plank, she builds a boat using the original planks, and voila! You now have two boats! Are they the same boat?

What's the point of this philosophical digression? The human body replaces its own cells regularly. Scientists at the Weizmann Institute of Science in Israel have investigated the specifics of how fast and to what extent cells are replaced. Firstly, they determined that about a third of our body mass is made up of fluid outside of our cells as well as solids, such as the calcium that gives bones structure. The remaining two thirds is made up of roughly 30 trillion human cells. Here are some fascinating numbers:

1. About 72% of the 30 trillion cells are fat and muscle, and they last about 12–50 years, respectively.

2. Blood cells of various types live for only 3 to 120 days.
3. The lining of the gut typically live less than a week.
4. Fat cells and bone elements live for a fairly long time, about 10 years.
5. Your tooth enamel is never replaced.
6. Parts of your brain don't appear to regenerate as you age, although the research on this may be showing that there is some change. Nevertheless, if there is regeneration, it is slow.
7. About 330 billion cells are replaced every day, meaning about 1% of all our cells. In 100 days, 30 trillion will have replenished – the equivalent of a new you!

You are like the Ship of Theseus! You are a vessel in which in 100 days, 30 trillion cells have been replaced by new ones. You have discarded all the old cells that were you. And so, are you constantly hating the new cells as they form? Or do you continue to hate the ones you have discarded?

The point is that when you think of this as an experiment in logic, the *you* that is the physical form is constantly changing so there is no constant you that you can hate. The element that feels stickier is that of thinking, and the constellation of thoughts that make you who you are. These are shaped by your biology, genetics, and experiences, and if you have had traumatic things happen to you, you can end up concluding that you are something loathsome; however, this is your brain attacking you with negativity and this can change, even if you don't believe it can.

Are You Bacteria?

Bacteria tend to have a negative reputation; however, here is a group of organisms, mostly bacteria that live in and around human tissues, and scientists call this the human microbiome. Some of these bacteria just co-exist with us, they go along for the ride but neither help nor hurt us. Yet others are essential for body functions, and we would die without them; for instance, the bacteria in the gut, and then of course, there are bacteria that cause significant illness. What is fascinating is that researchers (Sender et al. 2016) have calculated that there are slightly more bacterial cells, 39 trillion, than there are human cells, 30 trillion, in the human body. In other words, more than half of your total number of cells are bacteria. Many of them are an essential part of who we are, our self. Are we hating them as well?

The key point to this section is that when you say or think "I hate myself," remember that you are a vast network of many different components. Your self is made up of human-self elements such as your cells with human DNA, and non-human elements, which include bacterial cells and elements such as calcium, carbon, phosphorus, and so on. Some, like the essential bacteria or the calcium that makes up your bones, are critical for life, and cannot realistically be removed, but for most people who are reading this book, this is not the self that they mean when they say, "I hate myself." For them, the elements of self-hatred tend to be narrower than the vastness of the self and tend to have more to do with thoughts and emotions, and by being clear about exactly what you mean by the self, you take your first step in overcoming self-hatred.

In the next chapter we will see how self-hatred develops and how you came to learn, falsely, that it is a core part of how you are.

Part 2

Roots of Self-Hatred

Chapter 6

Where Does Self-Hatred Come From?

"No one is born hating another person because of the color of his skin, or his background, or his religion. People must learn to hate, and if they can learn to hate, they can be taught to love, for love comes more naturally to the human heart than its opposite."

—Nelson Mandela, *Long Walk to Freedom*

If we apply this profoundly compassionate wisdom to the concept of self-hate, here is what I would say: You are not born hating yourself because of who you are. You have to learn to hate yourself, and if you can learn to hate yourself, you can learn to love yourself, because love comes more naturally to the heart than the opposite.

So, how do people learn to hate themselves? I wanted to understand how people developed this sense of self, how they had learned to hate themselves, so I asked some patients, present and former, people I care deeply about, to think about this question and then share their reflections. I asked them to answer the questions that I outlined in Chapter 2. Here is what they have to say:

How Far Back Do You Remember Self-Loathing?

Answer 1: *"I remember having a lot of self-judgment in early elementary school, or even before. I think once I became aware that my level of anxiety was abnormal, is when the self-hatred started. I also think that it is important to say that I fell into patterns of comparing myself* *to my friends when I was really young, maybe as early as first grade, and I thought that they were prettier, or had nicer stuff, or had nicer parents, and then that I didn't deserve anything, which is definitely a big piece of where my self-loathing comes from."*

Answer 2: *"I don't have a memory of not feeling self-loathing and my earliest memories are exactly that. Maybe around the age of 4–5 and my memory is of hating myself and crying because I accidentally pushed on my mom the wrong way while trying to snuggle with her on the couch. She said 'ouch!' and I was so upset with myself for hurting her. Then, if I got in trouble, I would sit in my room and just lament about what an awful person I was. There is no 'before' with the self-loathing, at least in my memory. I always felt like I came off the assembly line defective."*

Answer 3: *"As far back as I can remember. When I try to remember a time in my life without chronic self-loathing, it did exist before I had to socialize and interact with the outside world (before elementary school). I think my self-loathing began to emerge during the early days of elementary school when it became apparent that socializing/mingling with peers was difficult for me and I began to feel like an outsider. My first suicide attempt at age 8 was brought on by my conviction that this world would bring me nothing but unhappiness."*

Answer 4: *"Honestly far back. I remember being so young thinking I was the worst person to exist. My family started going to family therapy when I was in fifth grade and the whole time, they would talk about what I did wrong that week. I would watch all my friends and think well their family does not need to go to family therapy because they are not bad kids. I was constantly compared to my 'perfect' brother. My earliest memories consisted of me lying in bed staring at my ceiling thinking 'God, maybe if I was dead people would finally care about me.' I specifically remember wondering if I were dead, 'What they would say about me?' 'Would they say they loved me?' 'Would they say they didn't even care?' I always concluded, who could care about a kid as bad as me?*

"It started around when I was eight or nine years old. When I was in fourth grade, I would fight a lot with my parents and my brother – he was the perfect child, he would never argue with them. I was also going to family therapy, which was a 'Shit on Me' show. So, after a while of my parents calling me a piece of shit or a bitch, I started believing I was a bad kid and there must be something wrong with me. I genuinely thought that I had a disorder or something that made it so I could not function properly because as a little kid what else would I think? Then when I was older, about 14, I was raped and blamed for it. At the time I was drinking and when people found out their first response became, 'well maybe if you hadn't drunk that much you wouldn't have gotten raped.' I thought, 'OK but he also did a bad thing.' But everyone continued talking to him and stopped talking to me. I mean, what do you conclude about yourself other than that you are worthless? This destroyed the small bit of self-compassion that remained in my brain. Who would love the girl that was over dramatic and blamed someone else for something she could have controlled. I mean it was nailed into my brain; how could I not think that?"

Answer 5: *"It feels like I was born this way.... I can't remember a time that I liked myself or felt anything other than pure hatred and disgust towards myself. You believe it is learned? If it is learned, how did I learn it so strongly from such a young age? People think that it started at the age of 12 when I was first sexually assaulted.... and then it happened again and again and that has been a great source of evidence I have for my belief that I am 1) fundamentally terrible and 2) disgusting. HOWEVER, my deep self-hatred began far before the age of 12.... so then what explains that? I think that it is the other way around. Bad things happened to me because I was bad."*

Answer 6: *"My self-hatred has grown and flourished as a result of the idea of failure. When I was really young, say about five or six, I had no notion of self-hatred, only the new excitement each day would bring. That all changed when I reached around sixth grade. I started* *to become self-conscious, hiding every part of me I could. My older sister, on the other hand, would wear all these cute, fashion-forward outfits and I would become envious that I could not get out of my own head to wear clothes like my sister wore. Even to this day, I wish I had the confidence to wear what my sister wears. This idea would lead to self-hatred because I would hate the person I was becoming and love the person my sister was becoming. Also, around this time, I started to become increasingly aware of my parents' arguments, and how they pertained to me. My mother would say things like my father was turning me into a monster. I would try to step up and defend my father or my sister from my mother's harsh words, but I only ever made things worse. This would lead to an immense amount of self-loathing because I felt that I was the problem in the family, and I needed to leave for the family dynamics to become better. I would constantly beat myself up, wondering why I couldn't be the perfect daughter my sister was. I also started to find empty wine bottles around the house that my mom hid. When she drank, her attitude would change completely, and not in a good way. My mother says she drinks because of my father, and he is made the villain. This idea of my father being the villain would make me feel as though I had failed as a daughter, and that I was not worthy of love. Also, around this time, my best friend taught me how to self-harm. He told me to tell no one. I agreed, not wanting to get him into any trouble. Soon thereafter, he gave me a suicide note. It was then when I realized I should have told someone, which only led me to hate myself for not telling someone about my friend's suffering; I concluded I was a horrible friend. By the time I processed what he gave me, he asked for the letter back. I nodded and gave it back to him. I realized that I failed at being a friend. I had the opportunity to help him, and I blew it.*

"It was then that I realized that I had failed on multiple fronts: I had failed as a daughter, as a friend, and as a person. All this self-hatred would be made worse during my freshman year of high

school. I started to compare myself to people on social media, wishing I looked like them. I started to restrict my eating to achieve my ideal body. I lost weight and I lost weight fast. Despite the weight loss, I still hated myself. I hated the way I looked and how much I had to lie to achieve weight loss. During the period of weight loss, I met a boy and found him to be the only positive in my life. Then, he broke up with me, because, and this is what he told me, he 'couldn't handle me.' That caused me to spiral even further down, and I concluded that I was unlovable, and definitely not worthy of any sort of affection. So, failed as a daughter, friend, person, and now as a girlfriend. I started to self-harm, and almost became addicted to it. Now, my self-harm isn't that extreme because I do not want to go to the hospital. My self-hatred, however, is still going strong. I only wear clothes that hide my body, my scars, and my cuts. During the summer, I don't even want to leave the house. I don't think I'm worthy of self-love because I'm an awful person. I have been nothing but a burden to those around me."

Answer 7: *"I have experienced the feeling of self-hatred towards specific parts of myself for as long as I can remember. Feelings of complete/total self-loathing since I was 12 years old. Originally, I only hated my inability to think things over before speaking or acting and I hated my inability to reach the impossible standard of perfection. But then I was severely bullied at school. It was constant and no one got it, and no one stood up for me. I didn't really show how I felt. I acted tough, but then I would go home and cry for a long time. I thought that I had to be all the things that people said, the things they called me. Since being bullied/belittled and having had my entire personality/physical appearance picked apart I've grown to despise every aspect of myself."*

Answer 8: *"As far back as I can remember. (I don't remember a time when I didn't experience self-loathing.)"*

Answer 9: *"As long as I can remember having a self-concept (5ish)."*

These are nine different people who share a common experience of self-loathing. They do not know each other, are not connected in any way, and they are people I have worked with over the past 20 years, and yet their narratives transcend time, geography, socio-economic group, any other demographic, although most of them are women. What stands out is that for all nine, aged between their late teens and early 30s, the experience of this immovable self-hatred starts very young, as young as kindergarten or earlier.

Many people who experience self-loathing do not remember a clear time when they loved themselves, or if they do, it was when they were very young. That's a long time to live with such a painfully distorted sense of self.

EXERCISE

To prepare for this exercise, if you can, try to get a photo of every birthday, and maybe even the day that you were born. Ideally you have one of each birthday and your actual birthday! So, if you are 18, you would have 19 photos. If you are 32 you would have 33 photos. This exercise works even if there are gaps, so don't worry if you don't have them all. Now print the photos and lay them side by side on the floor. Take a moment to really notice how much you've changed over time from a child to an adolescent to an adult.

For the reflection exercise: When did your self-hatred begin? Say you think that it was age five. Can you look at a photo of you aged five, or the photos after that, and honestly say that you hate that child? Can you have compassion for the child that suffered? Can you see that there is no permanent self to hate, that there is a person flowing and changing throughout a life? You are changing at every moment. Why do you carry self-hatred with you as if it were a permanent thing? Of course, one version of you leads to the next version of you, but you are also constantly changing, and carrying self-hatred with you is both unbearable and unnecessary.

EXERCISE

How did your self-loathing begin? How did the lessons in self-hatred begin? Who were your teachers?

____

____

____

____

____

____

____

How Does Self-Hatred Develop?

> "This negative self-talk is something you probably aren't even aware of, but it eats away at you bit by bit and erodes that self-confidence you need to tackle your anxiety."
>
> —Robert Duff

Patients find this question to be a difficult one, because it implies a "time before" self-hatred, and they can't always remember. Then, most can't think of a single incident that caused them to hate themselves, and in part, this is because they feel that they were born flawed.

One patient shared this reflection: "I can't recall one specific incident, but I do remember the feelings developing and intensifying over time. I think the feelings started from internalizing others' expectations of me from a young age, and establishing early on the core belief that my self-worth was directly tied to my ability to meet others' expectations and make them happy. I think that as a highly sensitive child, experiences of punishment (verbal/physical), violent anger, and intergenerational trauma affected me to a much greater degree than it affects most people."

Theory and Research

This reflection is clearly a considered idea, and likely has tremendous merit. I went to the research to see if there were studies that might help answer the question and it turns out that there are four main theories as to how persistent self-hatred develops and is then maintained. The first theory is the most evolved, and I will review it more comprehensively. The other three theories are less developed and researched.

THEORY 1: One of the people who has thought about this is Australian psychiatrist Roy Krawitz. He proposes that a combination of a person's *attitudinal emotional stance* along with shame leads to the evolution of self-hatred. Here is an example in plainer English. Let's say that you perceive that you are a bad person because you forgot a friend's birthday. You then experience self-contempt and self-criticism, which in turn makes you feel even worse about yourself. Your attitudinal stance is the belief that you are a bad person together with the self-criticism and self-judgment. This can lead to you being angry at yourself and feeling that you need to be punished.

Imagine a different attitudinal stance: "I forgot my friend's birthday. I am sad that I did and yet I have been so busy and exhausted at work that it simply escaped me. I am a good friend to her, and I will make it up by taking her out to dinner."

Most people who don't experience persistent self-loathing have a positive, or at least more neutral, attitudinal stance, and so even if there is some incident that they perceive as unfortunate or negative, they don't then pile on a critical self-assessment. Instead, they are able to maintain a balanced perspective and avoid letting life's inevitable negative experiences define their overall self-worth.

What Is My Attitudinal Stance?

> "Yes, Eleanor loathed herself and yet required praise, which she then never believed."
>
> —Hanif Kureishi

EXERCISE

Think of an example when you experience a negative interaction or outcome. For instance, a friend did not call you back, you got a B on a paper that you were expecting an A on, your boss gave you some feedback at work. Or even consider what to others may seem like a normal interaction with another person, say that you are in line to get a coffee and the line is moving very slowly when you need to get to work.

Describe the situation below:

MY EMOTIONAL/ATTITUDINAL RESPONSE:

What are the thoughts that you have about yourself in the above situation? Do I:

Self-criticize?

Self-judge?

Feel disgusted with myself?

Feel that I am a failure?

Catastrophize?

Feel that others don't take me seriously because I am not important?

ALTERNATIVE RESPONSES: Given that people who do not hate themselves may have been in exactly the same situation, but not bring self-critical attitudinal responses to the situation, can you:

Make a self-validating statement? (I really studied for the test. I did the best I could, and the subject is tough for me.)

Make a kinder, or at least more neutral, statement about yourself? (Just because my boss made some suggestions as to how I could be more productive, does not mean she hates me or that I am the worst employee ever.)

See this as a temporary setback in the course of a day? (My friend did not call me back and I am disappointed, and yet he is a good friend, and we are having dinner later on.)

Think of alternative reasons for the other person's behavior? (For instance, the barista may be new at her job, or have worked a double shift, or have complicated orders to fill.)

By practicing some of these alternative responses, you begin to cultivate a more balanced and self-caring perspective toward yourself. Not all negative outcomes are because you've done something wrong; and in fact, many of the negative outcomes in life are rarely exclusively your fault, even if you believe that they are. Practicing self-validation, making more accurate self-assessments, viewing setbacks as temporary, and considering alternative reasons for others' behaviors is another inroad to reducing self-hate. This approach not only helps in addressing and lessening the reaction to self-hate as a behavior but also fosters resilience and a healthier, more constructive, and adaptive self-image.

THEORY 2: A second possible path to the evolution of self-hatred was proposed by Dr. Rottraut Ille (2014) who suggested that self-hatred develops through the emotion of disgust. What her theory states is that a person has an intense desire to distance themselves from something that is disgusting, which in this case is themselves. There are some people who find aspects of themselves to be repelling, and then what they want is to get rid of the repelling thing.

Think of it this way. Imagine that you went out for a walk in your brand-new pair of designer sneakers, and you step on dog poop. You notice the emotion of disgust, and then immediately turn around and go home to wash the poop off the shoe with your garden hose. However, imagine that you were someone who, after having stepped in dog poop, believed that the whole shoe was tarnished forever and that you had to get rid of the shoes. For people who experience intense self-loathing, certain behaviors and traumatic childhood experiences make them feel disgusted in themselves as a whole, as if the traumatic experience has tainted their entire being. They feel repelled by the self that was misused and they want to get rid of it. They cannot see that their abusers perpetrated great psychological damage and feel instead that they did something wrong and that their abuse was deserved for being flawed.

Trigger Warning: If the event that caused you to experience self-disgust was childhood abuse and you have not yet addressed this, whether in therapy or elsewhere, writing about it now may trigger powerful feelings. If this happens, it is your brain and body's way of telling you that it is something you need to address. If the answer is too painful, skip this exercise until you can address it with a trusted person.

EXERCISE

Do you feel disgusted by yourself? When did the self-disgust start? Did something specific happen to trigger the feelings of self-disgust?

ANSWER:

____

____

____

____

____

THEORY 3: An idea that some colleagues and I have worked on is derived from the biosocial model that Dr. Marsha Linehan proposed when she developed the treatment known as dialectical behavior therapy (DBT) (1993). Her biosocial theory posited that chronic emotional dysregulation emerged from repeated transactions between a child's biological emotional vulnerability and an invalidating developmental environment (more about invalidation in the next paragraph).

Human babies are born with the innate capacity to attract the type of care that will ensure their survival. Think of the response that most people have to the announcement of a newborn child. Typically, there is a tremendous amount of care given to meet the child's every need, and this is true whether or not the child later turns out to be emotionally sensitive. As children develop, they will require varying degrees of emotional support in order to thrive. Some will be okay with a simple pat on the back, while others will only feel supported if their expression of emotional experience is validated.

If, as the child grows, they turn out to be more emotionally sensitive, the environment will need to be more attuned to their emotional needs than if they are less sensitive. But what happens if emotional needs are not only not met, but the child further experiences the rejection of who they are and the way they respond to the world. Linehan's theory said that pathology and the destruction of the sense of self were a direct consequence of this emotional sensitivity and rejection.

We will delve further into this in a few pages; however, in my clinical experience, which research supports, children who experience chronic invalidation feel more flawed, inadequate, have lower self-worth, and are at risk for developing mental illness. The iniquity of all this is that because their cognitive and emotional brain systems are in the midst of massive evolution, children conclude that they are to blame for the way they feel, and this is a perfect recipe for the development of self-hate. Compounding all of this, is that in an environment that feels unresponsive or dismissive to their needs, the maladaptive and self-destructive coping mechanisms act quickly to reduce emotional pain, so they are reinforced. Importantly, if a family system is aware of this dynamic, they can take advantage of the rapidly evolving cognitive and emotional development and through the practice of validation, begin to reverse the scarring effects of invalidation.

A Word About Invalidation

Linehan said that invalidation occurs when a person tries to communicate their private thoughts and experiences to others, and if this communication is met with erratic, unpredictable, rejecting, punitive, or extreme responses, the person interprets the response as being told that their experience is not valid. When these private experiences are trivialized or punished, it leaves the person feeling belittled, disregarded, flawed, and inadequate.

Thought Experiment on Invalidation

Imagine that you meet up with three friends. One has a bad headache, one had a terrible night's sleep and is exhausted, and the third is doing fine. You propose a five mile hike up a hill. Obviously, you cannot see someone else's headache, someone else's tiredness, or someone else's being fine. You would take their word that they are experiencing whatever they tell you they are experiencing. If, on the other hand, one had a broken leg, you would visibly see a leg in a cast, but private thoughts or emotional experiences are not visible to others.

Now imagine that you insist on going on the hike, telling them that it will be good for them. When they complain about the headache or being tired, you tell them that they are making a big deal over nothing and that they should have the same attitude as the third friend, the one who is fine and who is up for the hike. Your rejection of the first two friend's experiences would be invalidation. You would be trivializing, dismissing, or disregarding what they are saying. Even if your intention is well meaning – in this case, your desire to be with your friends, be outdoors, and get some exercise – from the point of view of the others, you are being invalidating. Imagine if instead you were exhausted and needed to sleep or had a splitting headache. What would it feel like to be told that you were making a big deal over nothing?

Invalidation has two primary characteristics. Firstly, it tells the other person that they are incorrect in the description, interpretation, or assessment of their own experience. Secondly, it attributes their experiences to socially unacceptable characteristics of personality traits. In the example, imagine that you said to your two friends who were struggling, "You two are just making excuses and being lazy."

Let's continue with this example. Imagine that the friend with the headache gets upset with you, an understandable response. You then label her as being negative, oversensitive, and simply refusing to adopt a more positive attitude. You might even think that she is being manipulative, wanting sympathy from others, simply because your plan to go for a hike with your three friends is being compromised. Any of the labels you apply to her would be invalidating of her, because unless you know the characteristics to be factually correct, you are dismissing her experience. So, failure, or any deviation from some socially defined acceptable behavior – in this case to go on a hike – is attributed to being lazy, lacking motivation, or not trying hard enough.

Developmental Invalidation

How does invalidation impact a sensitive child? Not all children are born with the same biological temperament. Some are more sensitive than others. If a child: (i) has a biological predisposition to being emotionally sensitive, meaning that they experience emotions intensely, frequently, because of seemingly trivial reasons, and then take a longer time than others to recover from the emotional experiences, and (ii) is met with chronic invalidation from caregivers and other significant people in their life, the child learns that they need to work a lot harder to get their emotional needs met. They may double down on their efforts to get approval and acceptance from others and try to behave in ways that others find acceptable, but when emotions run high, "appropriate behavior" can be difficult.

If the invalidation persists, the child internalizes the invalidation and believes that she must be to blame for her strong emotions and unacceptable behavioral responses. When this happens, it can lead to a persistent experience of shame, and then the belief that she is at fault for being who she is. Over time, her shame strengthens because she feels that she cannot control any of the emotions or behaviors that parents and others label as "bad."

To cope with the debilitating emotion of shame, many people then resort to behaviors that quickly bring down the intensity of the shame. Unfortunately, many of the behaviors that work quickly are maladaptive, even if they are effective in the short term. These behaviors include avoidance, self-harm, suicidal behavior, and in the long run tend to hurt the person using them because they don't address the underlying shame and invalidation. Further, the behaviors reinforce the belief that they are undeserving, flawed, and unlovable.

I asked a patient what she thought of the biosocial theory, and here are her thoughts:

> *"Psychologically it makes sense that early childhood experiences with caregivers would influence the development of self-loathing;*

HOWEVER, would this be further dependent on how sensitive the individual child is? It makes me question my own experience; I grew up with my older sister (older by a year and a half), but here's the thing: We had the same parents, we lived in the same household, with the same rules and the same encouragements.

"So how do you explain that my sister is genuinely the most self-loving confident person I have ever met? Yes, self-loathing is tied to my body image. My sister, on the other hand, is incredibly body neutral and has always eaten intuitively. She openly discusses the things that she likes about herself and very rarely is self-critical (especially not in a highly negative manner). As you know, that is not exactly how I turned out. How does this happen? We were raised by the same caregivers in the same environment. Obviously, I am aware that we are different people and therefore were sometimes treated differently by my parents (especially surrounding food/body stuff), but with that I wonder if I was simply treated differently because of the presence of my self-hatred, so then how did mine develop so strongly?"

This reflection leads to an interesting question. Why is it that two children born into the same family can experience their sense of self so differently? One hates themselves and the other does not. The developmental expert, Dr. Gabor Mate says: "No two children are raised by the same two parents." By this he means that when parents have a second child, they are different people than they were when they had their first child. Further, because children are different biologically, emotionally, and temperamentally, the way that the parents act toward different children is different. For instance, parents may be more reactive, critical, and invalidating toward a more emotional child and calmer, less judgmental, and more tolerant of their less reactive child.

EXERCISE

Think about the concept of invalidation. How often were you told that what you were feeling was wrong, or that you were making a big deal of things, or that you shouldn't be feeling what you were feeling? How often have you been told to "just get over" things?

ANSWER: Write down the ways in which you have been invalidated.

____

____

____

____

____

<u>THEORY 4:</u> A Psychodynamic Model to the Development of Self-Hatred in Borderline Personality Disorder

This theory might be a bit more difficult to understand because psychodynamic theory can feel complicated. The psychodynamic model as to the development of self-hatred is very different from that of the biosocial model of DBT. Psychodynamic theory and therapies focus and explore a person's longstanding beliefs and desires, and per the theory, these are caused by early life experiences and further that many of these causes are not in a person's awareness. In other words, the causes lie in the unconscious. Therefore, the construct of the self as one to be loathed would have its hidden roots in the depths of early childhood experiences.

The psychologist Margaret Singer (1977) proposed the idea that a person with borderline personality disorder (BPD) who experiences their very core as defective finds it nearly impossible to integrate different parts of themselves into a whole that makes sense to them. She said that this was especially true if those parts seem to conflict with each other. For instance, say that you are kind to others and then say something mean to a friend. For people with BPD, holding on to the idea that the "kind self" and the "mean self" coexist is a difficult task. Similarly, they also find it difficult to reconcile different parts of other people, making it very difficult to see others in anything but all-or-nothing ways.

What is the consequence of this struggle to integrate opposing ideas? For example, let's say that a loved one is angry that you left the kitchen a mess, but that they then offer to help you clean up and then express gratitude. For those who see themselves as defective, the show of anger and kindness in one person is confusing, and they find it hard to see how a person can have both of those qualities.

Margaret Mahler (1975), a psychiatrist and pediatrician interested in child development, suggested that difficulties in early developmental stages could lead to a sense of emptiness. She described a phase known as rapprochement, occurring between the ages of 15 and 24 months. During this phase, the increasingly mobile infant, who no longer needs to be carried around, recognizes that they are separate from their mother. Mahler argued that if the child fails to navigate this stage successfully and becomes uncertain about their separateness, it could lead to enduring anxiety and fear of abandonment, especially if the mother responds with impatience, irritation, or lack of availability. In this context, the child finds it difficult to reconcile both the negative and positive aspects of the mother, leading to a fractured attachment and a resulting sense of emptiness.

In a paper on emptiness, psychiatrist Stephen Levy (1984) defined this emptiness as the "loss of the normal background feeling tone guaranteed by the cohesiveness of internalized object relations." What this means is that the typical and predictable feeling of security that most children feel because they simply "know" that their "object," meaning caregiver, a reliably constant person, will respond predictably, is not what the person with BPD experiences. Levy suggested that the BPD child can't predict that their parent will be reliable because they haven't been. Because the BPD child is unable to integrate the various parental responses, the "good" and "bad" aspects of his mother, that the child would then struggle and try to identify only with the good or wanted parts of the mother and try to "repudiate" or "eliminate" the negative or unwanted parts.

Many people find these ideas challenging to grasp because they are not commonly aware of experiencing their parents in this way. With these psychoanalytic concepts in mind, the path to self-hatred can be understood as follows: the painful experience of emptiness, particularly common in patients with BPD (see Chapter 8), prevents the possibility of self-acceptance. This is because self-acceptance can feel repulsive and deeply anxiety-provoking, leading to thoughts like, "How can I accept a repulsive me?" When therapists encourage a more compassionate self-view, patients may fixate on their perceived defects, feeling fundamentally different and broken. This focus on their flaws perpetuates and intensifies their self-hatred.

The internal split between the desire to feel "normal" and the experience of feeling defective can lead to an unrelenting inner war between opposing sides of the self. One side wants to get better and recognizes all the hard work that it will require, and the other side simply wants immediate freedom from the pain of self-hatred, and in this context, suicide then can be understood as serving as the ultimate protection from such suffering. Again, suicide is never the right solution.

And so, through the lens of psychodynamic theory, self-hatred in BPD is essentially seen as an attachment disorder symptom. The self-loathing reflects the perceived rejections of an unwanted child and develops during early childhood. The rejection of the unwanted self is seen as an unconscious and adaptive defense mechanism in that by disowning the part of the self that was rejected, abandoned, abused, or seen as too emotional or sensitive, the wanted part of the self might be something appealing, even praiseworthy to family, friends, and partners. Unfortunately, without addressing this struggle in therapy, the internalized self-hatred leads to persistent and intolerable suffering, and then, and as proposed by all theories, the idea of suicide as the ultimate solution to ongoing suffering.

Here is the bottom line: All the patients who have shared their experiences with me have said that their self-loathing started in childhood. All the theories on the development of self-hatred suggest that the child internalizes a sense that they are defective, and this sense grows to infect aspects of the self. To me it matters less as to how it developed. Understanding why an egg breaks when it falls to a granite floor does not make it any less broken. Of course, it is useful to understand in that knowing that the seeds of self-hatred were planted by experiences not of your choice is important in self-validation. However the you that is self-loathing now is the you that you are and that is the person that needs help, and not the little girl or boy that experienced the trauma. You can have compassion for that child, and, going forward you can commit to stand up against toxic elements that infest the minds of other children, but your task now is to begin to undo the harm that the damaging experiences of your past created.

One Patient's Reflection on How Her Self-Hatred Developed

When I suggest to patients that self-hatred is learned rather than some flaw they are born with, it gets many of them thinking. One patient found this idea so novel that she decided to map out the development of her self-hatred, and she sent me the following email.

"It was like an epiphany and then the more I thought about it, the more I tried to put it all together so here goes:

Question: What are the biosocial aspects of the development of your self-hatred, step-by-step?

a. *Biological predisposition*

i. *I have a genetic vulnerability and epigenetic predisposition. For generations back on my mother's side there is mental illness, addiction, and trauma experienced by my mom, my grandmother, and as far back as we know.*

b. *Invalidation*

i. *Growing up, it seemed to me that my mom was the only one in our house who was allowed to have feelings. She was severely mentally ill and often had frightening emotional* *outbursts, and many of these were directed at me. All I can remember her telling me over and over was that I was to blame for her problems. Little things like leaving my school lunch at home when I was in third grade, would lead to her saying that I must want her to have a totally miserable life, that she should kidnap my younger sibling and leave and never come back, or that I made her to want to smash her face. I remember this phenomenon occurring as early as when I was about eight years old.*

c. *Increase in acceptance-seeking behavior*

i. *The only way to control my mom's outburst was for me to work very hard to placate her and help her regulate her feelings. I would talk her down by saying that I loved her and that I didn't mean to make her feel this way, and that I would be so careful in the future to make sure that I didn't do whatever I had done to upset her, like forget my school lunch, or whatever it was. When she felt guilty after the fact, she told me to tell her that she was a good mother, that I was in the wrong, and that her reactions didn't make her a bad person. In between outbursts, I would go to extreme lengths to try to keep her happy and in a good mood. These efforts to increase the acceptability of my behaviors and existence were largely fear-based, although some of it also came from a want to be loved and accepted. I mean who doesn't want her mom to love her?*

d. *More invalidation*

i. *Despite my best efforts to keep my mom happy and calm, the outbursts would always continue to happen. As I got older, I began to try less to control her and instead would wait for her to be the bigger person or would try to be honest about the impact on me. These would only make her more upset and worsen her sense that she was the victim. I once told her that her behavior and the way she acted like a toddler made me feel like I didn't have an actual mom. Her immediate response* *was, 'that's the meanest thing anyone has ever said to me.' There was no reflection on the events leading to the outburst, or validation of my experiences. She experienced me sharing my experience as a personal attack on her, with her the victim and me the villain.*

e. *Internalization*

i. *But nothing ever changed, and over time, I began to think that maybe she was right, and I began to blame myself for my mom's behavior. I often regretted the way that I reacted, thinking that if I hadn't instigated her and egged her on at times, or if I had done a better job calming her down, then my childhood would've been less traumatic and that I wouldn't be so fucked up as an adult.*

f. *Shame*

i. *I feel intense shame around how I acted around my mother and about who I am as a person.*

g. *Reinforced behaviors*

i. *Engaging in self-harm, compulsive skin picking, suicide plans and attempts, and eating behaviors such as restricting and purging bring me even more shame and reinforce my feelings that I am a disgusting and messed up person and that I deserve for bad things to happen to me.*

h. *Self-hatred*

i. *My experiences, the shame that I feel surrounding them, particularly because they started at such a young age, and the mental illness and maladaptive behaviors that have resulted from them have fundamentally influenced my identity and self-concept. I feel as though I am disgusting, crazy, manipulative, incapable of doing anything meaningful, and not worthy of love or good things. At my core, I deeply hate myself and my actions and often think that I would be doing a favor to the world if I were to end my life."*

As this reflection demonstrates, the patient is neither responsible for her mother's mental illness nor is there anything she can do, or could have done, about it. But not understanding this at a young age led to the development of maladaptive behaviors and self-hate. The repeated invalidation and the impossibility of meeting her mother's emotional needs fostered a profound sense of inadequacy and self-loathing, shaping her identity and mental health in deeply negative ways. Her mother's behaviors were never her fault, and it wasn't until she was given this exercise that we were able to unpack this insight. She told me that by breaking it down in this way, that seeing how it evolved, helped her soften her stance toward herself, and perhaps it is an exercise you would find useful.

Chapter 7

Could It Be Temperament or Biology?

A few months ago, I received an email from a therapist who told me that she had watched one of my videos on overcoming self-hatred. She said that she found it to be conceptually useful, and that my focus on development and the path from early childhood experiences was clearly articulated. She then asked me something I had not considered: "Could self-hatred be biological or genetic?" In other words, could self-hatred be inherited, or could certain biological factors predispose a person to self-hatred? This is an excellent question, and I turned to the research literature. There is no research that shows a genetic or temperamental component to self-hatred, however there was one study that combined some of the topics that we have previously reviewed, and hints at the possibility that there may be some genetic and biological risk factors.

TRIGGER WARNING: Throughout this book, there are both personal accounts of, and research findings on, suicide. For people who struggle with suicidal ideation, reading these can bring the thoughts to the front of their mind. You might be sick of hearing me repeat myself, but SUICIDE IS NOT THE ANSWER. These personal accounts and research findings underscore the pressing need to address all the factors that are risk factors for suicide.

In the study (Smith et al. 2012) that examined the environmental and genetic contributions of suicidal behavior among male twins, the researchers pointed out that all previous studies on suicidal behavior had found that genetics accounted for between 40% and 50% of suicidal behavior, and that although this meant that there was a strong genetic influence on suicidal behavior, psychological and environmental factors accounted for the remaining 50–60%. In reviewing the psychological elements at the core of the Interpersonal-Psychological Theory of Suicide (IPTS), there are three causal factors that heighten the risk of suicide:

1. Perceived burdensomeness: This occurs when you come to the erroneous conclusion that your death is worth more to others than your life is.
2. Failed belongingness: This refers to feelings of loneliness and the perception that no one cares about you.
3. The acquired capability for suicide: This refers to a fearlessness about death and physical pain, a capability that develops over time through repeated exposure to painful and/or fear-inducing experiences.

The idea of the impact of biology resonated deeply with one of my patients, a person with borderline personality disorder (BPD) and an eating disorder, who shared the following:

> *"I got diagnosed with my primary illness, a genetic connective tissue disease, when I was 20. Around this time, I was also diagnosed with a number of comorbidities that required significant intervention. When I was 21, my mobility began to decline significantly, and I sometimes required the use of a cane or wheelchair. At this point, through therapy, I was better at accepting help from my dad, but I felt immense guilt in accepting it, and developed a severe burdensomeness complex. I felt bad that my dad had a defective child, and like my physical limitations were annoying and embarrassing for him. I felt that he would not want to be seen in public with me, that the extra time and care it took me to navigate my physical environment was a waste of his time, and that he did not deserve the psychological burden of having to worry about me and my health.*
>
> *"During the period of diagnosis and worsening of my physical health, my self-hatred changed and increased significantly due to the phenomena described above. I felt that my body was*

annoying, defective, useless, and a burden to my family and society. This, in combination with the way my disability affected my social life and sense of belongingness as a child, has had a significant effect on my self-hatred, suicidality, and use of maladaptive coping skills, such as self-harm and eating disorder behaviors. There was a significant correlation between the acute worsening of my mobility and one of my most significant eating disorder relapses, and then, when this worsened my self-hatred, suicide was the only thing that made sense, but of course, I never acted on it, otherwise I wouldn't be here to tell you about it. But it is something I want you to think about because you are interested in self-hatred and that is not to forget the biological impact of pain and chronic illness."

The IPTS theory states that in order for someone to die by suicide, they have to desire suicide. Then, when (i) perceived burdensomeness and (ii) failed belongingness are felt simultaneously, these experiences create a powerful desire for suicide. Further, if a person has (iii) the capability and means to complete suicide, the combination of these three factors put the person at very serious risk for completing suicide.

What the researchers hypothesized was that the acquired capability for suicide had to have strong genetic components because it involves pain tolerance and fearlessness when it comes to the idea of death. The ability to tolerate high levels of pain and the fearlessness of death results from the repeated experiences of, and exposure to, pain. Previous research has shown that the ability to tolerate pain has a strong genetic component.

Pain and Suicide

Here is an interesting, and seemingly contradictory finding: On the one hand, people who experience chronic physical pain are two times more likely to make a suicide attempt (Calati 2015). On the other hand, patients who self-injure, by, for example, cutting, and don't feel pain, are at higher risk of suicidal behaviors (Van Orden 2010). According to theories that look at suicidal ideation to suicidal action, only people who possess high enough pain tolerance are at the highest risk of making a lethal or near-lethal suicide attempt (Klonsky 2015). This is because for people contemplating suicide, they have to be able to tolerate enduring pain during the suicide attempt. Many people I see who have thought of suicide have told me that they won't make an attempt because they are afraid of the pain.

For people I have worked with who have made suicide attempts, the idea of pain is less of a concern. As one patient told me: "I can tolerate a lot more pain than most people. It started when people used to hurt me. I learned how to deal with it. Pain does not scare me." So, what explains the seeming contradiction that people who experience chronic pain are more likely to make an attempt, and those who self-injure who don't feel pain are also more likely to make an attempt? The answer is that people who self-injure often do so during states of heightened emotional pain, and that when they are in emotional pain, physical pain is not experienced as painful, or at least not as painful. For the same people who self-injure, when they are not in emotional pain, and they were to cut themselves, or they cut themselves accidently, they do feel physical pain. So, the seeming contradiction is solved by recognizing that whether a person experiences high levels of physical or emotional pain, or both, if they are able to tolerate those high pain states, they are at much higher risk for suicide.

Returning to the Smith study, the researchers expected that beyond the high pain tolerance, that environmental factors would contribute significantly to a failed sense of belongingness, and that this was because of the absence of reciprocally meaningful relationships. They also expected that these environmental factors would lead to their perceived burdensomeness. There is another seeming contradiction in the study: If a person does not believe that they belong, then how can they feel that they are a burden? One clinician asked me: "How is it that a person does not feel that anyone cares about them, and yet they feel that they are a burden to others? How can someone be a burden if no one cares about them?"

I explained it this way: Imagine that you live at home, and you feel that no one in your family cares about you, that is the lack of belongingness. But yet you are using your family's resources, their money, their food, their time, and so on. So, this person that feels that they are uncared for, further feels that they are a burden to their family. Both of these conditions can be true at the same time.

Smith's team concluded that in order to reduce suicide risk, failed belongingness and burdensomeness had to be the focus of therapy. This was more important than focusing on whether a person was capable of suicide, because feeling disconnected and burdensome are more likely to change than the biological component of pain tolerance.

Although this does not directly address the question of whether self-hatred could be biological or temperamental, it does consider that some experiences that people who hate themselves have, such as an ability to tolerate significant emotional pain, could have biological elements.

EXERCISE

Do you feel connected to others including your family and friends? Do you feel as if you are a burden to others? Write about your experiences with connectedness and burdensomeness and the impact of these on your self-hatred.

ANSWER:

____

____

____

____

____

____

____

____

REFLECTION: Reflect on your answer and consider the people who care about you and consider the way in which you are kind to others. How do you reconcile your answer with your true kindness and the appreciation that others have for you?

In the next few chapters, we'll look at mental health conditions and diagnoses where people experience a disproportionate level of self-hatred.

Part 3

Self-Hatred in Mental Health

Chapter 8

Borderline Personality Disorder (BPD) and Self-Hatred

This is not a book about borderline personality disorder (BPD), and if this chapter is not relevant to you, you can certainly skip it. Nevertheless, I include it because when compared to other mental illnesses, people with BPD experience higher levels of enduring self-loathing than in other mental health conditions, and so it is important to highlight. Also, in the past, there were no dedicated treatments for BPD and so it was considered a difficult disorder to treat. This meant that people with BPD endured their symptoms, including self-hatred, for many years. Today, new treatments for BPD have had a significant impact on reducing the suffering that BPD causes. Self-hatred is not one of the diagnostic criteria for BPD, and yet, despite its significant impact on causing severe emotional pain, it remains the most significant unaddressed experience in BPD (Wilner et al. 2024).

In this chapter I have NOT included exercises. It is very important that you not self-diagnose; however, if many of these criteria seem to apply to you, I recommend that you consult with a mental health specialist, especially one with experience with BPD.

For the past 25 years, I have dedicated my clinical practice to working with a predominantly BPD population. Many of my patients, past and present, often endorse the symptom of self-hatred when I ask them about it, and the sense of core self-hatred is significantly profound in those who have also experienced significant childhood maltreatment. Although contemporary treatments for BPD don't include the targeting of self-hatred, it is my hope that these treatments and some of the ideas in this book can be integrated in order to tackle not only the standard and traditional diagnostic symptoms of BPD, but self-hatred as well.

What Is BPD?

Although BPD is not a condition that most people have ever heard of, it occurs far more commonly than many other psychiatric disorders and is very well known in mental health circles. Formal research shows that BPD occurs in somewhere between 2% and 6% of the general population. In outpatient clinics, nearly 20% of people have BPD, and on inpatient psychiatric units, almost 40% of patients have the condition.

In recent times there have been some high-profile cases with celebrities disclosing the diagnosis of BPD. This led to a significant increase in awareness, and in an informal survey of popular media sites, the hashtag BPD (#BPD), showed up more than four billion times; the more commonly known bipolar disorder had more than two billion views.

Someone with BPD typically has difficulty in the following five areas of functioning. They can struggle with: (i) regulating their emotions, (ii) maintaining stable relationships, (iii) managing impulsivity and self-destructive behaviors, (iv) experiencing significant distortions in the way they think, and (v) not having a consistent sense of self.

These are not transient experiences, but instead ones that happen regularly. One of the main differences between the symptoms of BPD and the ordinary difficult moments of life is the way that the symptoms impact a person's overall functioning. For instance, many people can have bad days, feeling low or irritable. For people with BPD, when the emotions engulf them, getting anything done feels nearly impossible. On the other hand, like with everyone else, when they are in a good mood, life is easier. For many people with BPD, behavior and completion of tasks is mood dependent. As you might imagine, mood-dependent behavior can significantly impact quality of life.

Here are the criteria of BPD. You may not relate to every one of them, but a few may resonate. For a person to be diagnosed with BPD, they need to meet at least five of the following nine criteria. It has been calculated that there are 256 different combinations of these symptoms that can meet criteria for BPD, and so even if you meet someone else with BPD, it is theoretically possible that you share only one symptom in common.

1. **People with BPD are terrified that they will be abandoned by the people most important to them, and this fear exists whether the threat of abandonment is real or not.** This means that at times, the person with BPD could in fact be experiencing the loss of a close friend or romantic partner, but in other circumstances, the fear of loss is only real in their mind. The manifestation of this fear can become problematic when in their desperation not to be abandoned, they do behaviors that can appear excessive, or even frantic, in order for the feared abandonment not to occur. Of course, no one wants to be abandoned, especially not by the people we care about. For people with BPD, this fear can be so unbearable that their thoughts turn to suicide.

   When the person with BPD also experiences severe self-loathing, the fear of abandonment can seem so real because they can't imagine that another person could love someone like them. What can then sometimes happen is that the person with BPD acts in frantic ways, or as one of my patients put it, "I reek of desperation," in order to prevent abandonment from happening. These frantic behaviors can include actions such as making constant phone calls, sending hundreds of texts, pleading for reassurance that the other won't leave, or showing up at irregular times at their home or place of work. When all else fails, the person with BPD might at times feel that the fear of abandonment is so unbearable that they turn to self-destructive behaviors including self-injury and suicide attempts. Sometimes, these have the effect of eliciting care from others, and then the problem is that these behaviors are reinforced. This means that if these behaviors lead to others expressing care, they may then repeat the behaviors whenever they feel that the other is going to leave.

   Here is where these frantic efforts eventually backfire. If you can imagine someone calling you or texting you incessantly or showing up at your home or place of work all the time, or making suicide attempts, you can imagine that these behaviors may be too much for you and wear you down. And so, the problem with these maladaptive behaviors is that they can lead to the very outcome that the person with BPD fears. Even if the loved one had no intention of leaving, they often experience these excessive behaviors as needy, clingy, and intrusive and then conclude that the relational demands are just too much, and then determine that leaving is best for their own mental health.

2. **People with BPD experience intense and unstable relationships that swing between idealizing other people.** For example, believing the other to be perfect on some occasions, and then at times devaluing the very same person and not seeing any good in them at all. This is explained by an important concept known as splitting that comes from psychodynamic theory, the type of therapy that was made famous by Freud. Splitting is considered an unconscious defense mechanism, where a person experiences polarized views of themselves or others. Splitting manifests with the person with BPD idealizing their partner at one moment and then devaluing them at another. The theory is that splitting allows the person with BPD to tolerate intense negative views about themselves and other people by seeing them as either good or bad, but not both good and bad. The problem is that when the person only experiences the negative self, they end up experiencing the darkest, least likeable part of who they are and this can lead to self-hatred.

3. **People with BPD can experience a marked, unstable, and persistently fluctuating sense of self, or even a lack of any solid sense of self at all.** This means that they recognize that their goals, employment dreams, religious beliefs, academic aspirations, gender identity or sexual preference and so on, are in a state of constant flux. Their sense of self can feel shattered or fragmented. One of my patients told me: *"I feel like I am a jigsaw puzzle, but that the pieces don't make up the picture on the box and it's worse,'cause I feel that someone just threw a bunch of pieces from different puzzles into the box, so I will never be complete."* One of the ways I see this manifest is that the person with BPD looks around and sees their peer group

graduate college in four years, certain of their career aspirations, seeing them in relatively stable relationships. The person with BPD on the other hand might take time off, switch majors, switch colleges, decide on one career path and then feel very dissatisfied with the choice, and then struggle with finding a partner or with whether they even want a partner. The problem is not that people with BPD struggle with making decisions, but rather that they don't have a stable sense of who they are and don't know where or how, or even if, they fit in. Feeling like such a "misfit" can fuel the self-hatred.

4. **People with BPD experience episodes of impulsive and potentially risky behaviors.** These can include gambling or spending sprees, reckless driving, unprotected, even dangerous, sex with multiple or unknown partners, binge eating and purging, or drug misuse. These behaviors typically serve the function of reducing the intensely painful emotions that come with feelings of loneliness. At times people with BPD say that they feel numb and so these behaviors can also function to help them feel alive or connected to others. The impulsivity can also include suddenly quitting a good job or ending a healthy relationship.

People with self-hatred can feel so bad about themselves that they feel that they deserve whatever happens to them. One patient told me about a relationship that they had established with another man. *"I met him online. It's kind of fun, and I like that he likes to slap me during sex, but recently he started punching me in the face,"* he told me. I was shocked on hearing this and asked him to tell me more about it, especially knowing his past and his childhood abuse. I asked him why he persisted in such a hurtful relationship. *"I am worthless, and I deserve it,"* he continued. *"And it's not all bad, and who else could I get?"* Self-hatred can lead the person with BPD to engage in impulsive and potentially dangerous behaviors because the person feels that they deserve it, or because they feel so unlovable that they will accept anyone, no matter how hurtful the person is.

5. **Suicidal behavior and self-injurious behavior, such as cutting, are both a hallmark of BPD.** BPD is a condition with a high suicide rate, although fortunately with new treatment methods, the suicide rate is decreasing. When people with BPD suffer emotionally, the suffering can be so unbearable that suicide seems like a viable solution. Alternatively, people with BPD self-injure as a way to reduce their emotional pain, or alternatively because they feel numb, or because they feel that they should be punished.

   As I mention throughout this book, and as research shows, self-hatred is a significant risk factor for suicide in people with BPD, and in part it is because they feel that they are a burden to the people in their lives and to the world as a whole. I can't overstate enough just how wonderful most people with BPD are. Most people with BPD are highly sensitive people who struggle with how they see themselves and would often want to remove themselves from situations rather than hurt others.

   I'll repeat myself here, as I do throughout the book. Suicide is not the answer to self-hatred or emotional suffering. If you have BPD and can learn to see how wonderful you are, you will see that suicide makes no sense. Many of the people who helped me think about the experience of self-loathing, those who have lived with self-hatred for years, and who believed that it would never change, are now professionally successful people in healthy relationships and whose struggles are those of ordinary life, and ones that they now feel are manageable.

6. **People with BPD can often feel as if they are on an emotional roller coaster, and experience frequent and intense mood episodes.** These are typically triggered by interactions with other people or by persistent negative self-talk. Although many people can notice mood changes throughout the course of a day, for people with BPD these mood shifts can be triggered by events and thoughts that to others seem trivial. For instance, maybe someone didn't say good morning. Maybe a friend did not return a call. Maybe a boss

questioned a decision. Although these incidents may be annoying or mildly upsetting to others, to the person with BPD these events can cause emotional storms and if they don't know how to manage the emotions, the consequence can be significant emotional and behavioral reactions. These reactions can also be triggered by negative inner dialogue including thoughts of self-hatred, self-criticism, and unkind thoughts.

For people who don't understand how something trivial might elicit a strong reaction, let's take a look at a peanut allergy. People who aren't allergic to peanuts can eat peanuts all day long, completely unaware of how many products even use peanuts as an ingredient. However those who are allergic can have a massive reaction even on exposure to a single peanut or peanut ingredient. For others with extreme allergy, a single peanut can cause death. Using this analogy, it is important to remember people react differently; some seemingly small rejection or criticism to the person with BPD can lead to a big emotional reaction in the way that one peanut can lead to a big physical reaction in the person who is allergic to peanuts.

7. **People with BPD describe feeling empty or disconnected or lonely much of the time.** This feeling of emptiness can seem confusing to those who don't experience it. It has to do with not feeling connected and presents as a deep longing or yearning for someone to fill a void in their lives. For people with BPD, it is not the absence of people that makes them feel lonely. They can feel lonely even in a crowd, if there is no one person they feel connected to. Many people will have the experience of feeling disconnected and lonely in certain situations such as being dropped off at college on their first stay, starting at a new high school, moving to a new city, and so on. However, most people then make connections, and they feel less lonely. Because people with BPD experience emotions and relationships so intensely, they often have the experience of feeling misunderstood or unable to be understood. Imagine being dropped into a jungle village where you don't speak the language, you don't

eat the food, and you don't understand the culture. Imagine how alone and strange you would feel. People with BPD often feel that they are a stranger in their world because they don't completely understand others' reactions and they are confused that others don't see their perspective. In my analogy, it is even more complicated for people with BPD because they don't have to imagine a jungle village. They actually speak the language and get the culture. However, what others often miss is the intense sense of disconnection and loneliness that people with BPD experience, which can be difficult to express in words. Because of this, they often feel defective, experience self-hatred and the understandable deep wish that they could "be like other people."

8. **People with BPD often experience excessive and intense anger, can appear to rapidly lose their temper, an in extreme situations, this can lead to destruction of property and on occasion, physical fights.** There can be hurtful verbal attacks filled with sarcasm and cruelty aimed at other people. The problem with the behaviors associated with the anger, other than the obvious, is that physical and emotional attacks are rarely consistent with the person's value system. People with BPD recognize that verbal attacks can temporarily feel good but soon they feel profound guilt and shame, emotions that can magnify any pre-existing self-hatred. Further, these types of anger-based attacks often leave people with BPD feeling that these attacks are further evidence that they are worthless, and not deserving of love.

9. **People with BPD, particularly if they have experienced the trauma of physical, sexual, or emotional abuse, often experience dissociation, which is the sense of not feeling real, or feeling that the rest of the world is not real.** In moments of intense emotion, which can be triggered by memories of trauma, their body feels disconnected from their emotions, and it can feel as if body and emotions are separate entities. When I speak to people who have been victims of abuse, especially when it happened in

childhood, they tell me that the connection to self-loathing is that they feel that they must be flawed or worthless because what else explains how easily they were misused or discarded, especially if the other was someone who was supposed to care for them.

Another distortion of reality that can occur is the feeling of paranoia. Paranoia tends to show up during moments of stress and can include feeling that others have evil intentions toward you, that others are talking about you, that everyone has negative thoughts about you, or that they are plotting against you.

Understanding BPD and its common symptoms provides insights into the challenges faced by those with the condition. People with BPD struggle with emotional instability, regulating interpersonal relationships, and a fluctuating sense of self, all of which can contribute to feelings of self-hatred. These symptoms create the type of emotional pain and self-hatred that can feel unbearable.

Again, it is important to recognize that this chapter is not meant for self-diagnosis. Instead, its purpose is to illuminate the relationship between BPD and self-hatred, highlighting the importance of compassionate and informed support for those affected. By better understanding these connections, we can foster greater empathy and develop more effective strategies for helping navigate the challenges. It is important to note, professional help and therapy can make a significant difference in managing BPD and finding some relief from accompanying self-hatred. Even though self-hatred is a very common experience in BPD, self-hatred is learned, and a false conclusion. If you have BPD, this book will address ways to overcome self-loathing.

Chapter 9

Other Psychiatric Diagnoses and Self-Hatred

We have just reviewed borderline personality disorder (BPD) as a mental health condition with significant self-loathing, but it is certainly not the only diagnosis that causes self-hatred to integrate itself into the self. In this chapter we'll review other conditions where self-hatred can show up as a part of the clinical profile and where self-hatred impacts a person's functioning. Again, in this chapter, I will not assign exercises related to self-diagnosis, and any exercises are there for the purpose of reflection, and not diagnosing yourself. If you feel strongly that these diagnoses apply to you, as with my recommendation in the previous chapter, it is important that you speak to a mental health specialist to receive, or rule out, a specific diagnosis.

Eating Disorders

Recently, a colleague asked me if I would help her out on her residential unit. Whereas I work predominantly with people who have BPD, her unit treats people with eating disorders (EDs). Although many of my patients struggle with eating, until recently I was less familiar with EDs as a diagnostic category. During the time I spent working with her I developed a more complete knowledge of formal EDs such as anorexia, binge-eating disorder, and bulimia.

Almost all of the patients on the unit were dissatisfied with themselves and because of my interest in helping people who struggle with self-loathing, beyond questions on eating behaviors, I asked the patients more about how they saw themselves and their self-image. Some of the patients told me how the dissatisfaction with their bodies had become a hatred of their bodies and then for some, that this body-hatred had morphed into an overall self-hatred.

With every new interview, I discovered that many patients with EDs had high levels of self-hatred. It got me thinking: Given that self-loathing can appear so enduringly in people with BPD and now, it appeared, EDs, I wondered about the comorbidity, or simultaneous presence, of EDs and BPD. Research shows that about 54% of people with BPD also have a history of an eating disorder (Khosravi 2020). About 25% of people with anorexia nervosa and 28% of people with bulimia nervosa have comorbid BPD.

What about research on core beliefs in EDs? A study (Fairchild and Cooper 2010) examined core belief items in 500 female participants. The participants were also asked to complete self-report measures of eating disorder symptoms, depression, anxiety, and self-esteem. The researchers found that people who scored high on self-loathing were more likely to be diagnosed with a formal eating disorder, while those who scored high on feelings of abandonment and deprivation were more likely to have anxiety and depression diagnoses. The researchers concluded that negative core self-beliefs relevant to those with an eating disorder were a multidimensional construct and that self-loathing as a core belief merited further research and clinical attention. I couldn't agree more, and yet sadly, this recommendation has gone unheeded by many of us who work as therapists.

Self-blame and eating disorders: In research (Petersson et al. 2021) that looked into factors that predicted remission from EDs in a group of 60 patients, 41 of them attained remission. What is startling is that of all the possible reasons that they attained remission, the only significant predictor of diagnostic remission after nine years was initial levels of self-blame. When the researchers drilled down on the results, they found a significant difference between those with binge-eating disorder, most of whom had recovered, and those with anorexia nervosa, who had the poorest outcome, where slightly more than half of patients recovered after nine years. The researchers hypothesized that because eating disorder behaviors are sometimes used to regulate negative emotions and unwanted thoughts, and further because eating behaviors subjectively improve a person's self-perceived flaws (for instance if they felt they were overweight, starving their body made them thinner) then because they temporarily feel better, self-blame reinforces the eating behavior. "If by starving myself I am getting rid of the thought that I am fat, and then when I starve myself I lose weight, then that's a good thing." In other words, if a person is having negative thoughts about themselves, and then feel that they are physically flawed, by beating themselves up and blaming themselves for the negative thoughts and flaws, they "try harder" in their disordered eating behavior.

Because self-blame is a symptom related to self-hatred, exposing the ways in which it can hijack healthier thinking processes allows for a more direct approach to targeting the self-blame as a symptom. The authors of the study concluded: "Viewed in a clinical context, focusing on self-criticism may be essential for achieving long-term recovery from ED. Indeed, initial negative self-image (i.e., high levels of self-blame and self-hate) can be reduced to normal levels after ED treatment. The road to long-term recovery in ED may, therefore, not just require symptom-focused interventions, but also therapeutic techniques that increase self-compassion, the opposite of self-blame."

While there is much more research to be done, this study highlights the critical role of self-blame in the persistence of eating disorder behaviors. This research mirrored my experience in working with patients with EDs. By recognizing that self-blame, tied closely to self-hatred, can undermine healthier thinking patterns, there is an identified need for therapeutic techniques that focus on reducing self-criticism and promoting self-compassion, in addition to addressing the symptoms of EDs. This comprehensive approach could be key to achieving long-term recovery and improving the overall well-being of people with EDs.

Lived Experience

When I asked a patient about how her self-hatred and her eating disorder were connected, this was her insight. *"My anorexia is closely tied to my self-hatred. They both feed into each other in a vicious cycle. Self-hatred severs my mind-body connection and breaks my sense of trust and respect toward my body. Restriction and exercise then become a means of controlling my body and punishing myself for having needs and taking up too much space, physically and metaphorically. My anorexia also feeds into my self-hatred because while my ED serves a vital function in my life, and I am often ambivalent about letting go of it, and so I feel immense shame around my ED. I feel that I don't have a valid reason for having an ED, and I am ashamed of the decisions I've made in service of my ED that don't align with my values, and so how can I love the person I am?"*

Another patient said this about self-hatred and anorexia: *"For me it's comparisons. Comparisons definitely impact my self-hatred because they almost always leave me feeling inadequate, invalid, and incompetent. For instance, when I compare my body to someone else's body, it always amplifies my hatred toward my appearance because I see others as looking better than me. At the same time, the fact that I'm having these comparison thoughts that don't align with my values causes immense shame, which further perpetuates my self-hatred."*

These testimonials further reinforce that self-hatred needs to be assessed in patients with EDs.

Body Dysmorphic Disorder

> "If you're thin enough, then you don't have that ass that everybody wants. But if you have enough weight on you to have an ass, your stomach isn't flat enough. It's all just f—ing impossible. It causes you to go into a real shame/hate spiral."
>
> —Taylor Swift

On the eating disorder unit, many of the patients also struggle with poor body image and body dysmorphic disorder (BDD). Although many patients with EDs have poor body image, not everyone with poor body image has a formal eating disorder even if they have disordered eating. What I discovered was that many people who struggled with very poor body image also had core self-loathing. When they described the self-hatred, it appeared similar in presentation to the group of patients that I typically treat. Even though there was some overlap as to the development of the self-hatred, there were also some differences. Nevertheless, the self-hatred appeared to be just as impactful in their lives.

Here is what one of the patients told me: *"I hate my body, and it has caused me to have terrible self-esteem. I spend so much time looking at my body every time I walk by a window, every time I am in the bathroom and seeing myself in the mirror. It's almost as if looking at myself so many times will cause it to change or will motivate me to do something to change myself. I think that I am so gross, and then I think that I am so ugly, and then I wonder who could ever want someone so fat and ugly. And then, the more I like someone, the more I obsess about what they think about me, and what they think about how I look. It also really impacts me with how I dress because some of my clothes make me look so fat. I tried to diet, and I restricted what I ate, and once I was so thin and people told me I looked great, but then I couldn't go out to dinner because I was terrified that I would gain weight. I was so hungry and miserable, and then someone told me that I was like a skeleton, and then I started to eat, but then no one told me I looked good. It led to a cycle of self-loathing that has not ended."*

The Concept of Body Image

Body image is not an objective concept. While a person's physical attributes – such as height, weight, and eye color – are measurable, body image is a multi-dimensional construct. It affects everyone, whether they have a healthy or unhealthy perception of their body, and is influenced by cultural trends, nationality, race, ethnicity, and other factors. The components of body image include:

- **Cognitive:** This involves all the thoughts and beliefs you have about your body.
- **Perceptual:** This refers to how you perceive the size and shape of your body and its parts.

- **Affective:** This encompasses the feelings and emotions you have about your body.
- **Behavioral:** This includes the actions you take to examine, alter, or conceal your body.

Understanding the complexity of body image is crucial for creating a healthier relationship with your own body. Fostering a less negative body image involves being kinder to yourself and supporting developing a balanced view of your body. Ultimately, embracing the multi-dimensional nature of body image will lead to greater self-acceptance.

EXERCISE

If you struggle with poor body image, write down the ways in which you:

i. Think about your body, and the beliefs you have about your body,

ii. Perceive your body's shape and size,

iii. Feel about your body, meaning the emotions that show up for you when you think about your body,

iv. The behaviors that you do to check your body or change the shape of your body.

Related to poor body image is the diagnosis of BDD. With BDD, the person struggles with an over-emphasis or excess focus on a specific body part, which is different from an overall unhappiness with their entire body shape or size in people with poor body image. For people with BDD, life can be debilitating. You focus intensely on your appearance and body image, spend hours in front of mirrors, grooming yourself, checking for the tiniest imperfection or seeking reassurance from others. Your perceived flaw and the repetitive checking of these flaws can cause you significant distress and impact your ability to function.

One patient with BDD was predictably late for our therapy appointments. *"I just can never find the exact outfit that will make me feel perfect.*

I have 100s of outfits and I spend all my money on them, but none of them are just right." I knew that she really wanted to work on this and wanted to have extra sessions to address it, however she was nearly paralyzed by her weekly outfit indecision. I worked with her to modify the "tardiness to therapy" behavior using reinforcement principles. Because I knew that she wanted extra time, I told her that if she could wear sweats and show up on time for a month, that I would increase her sessions to twice a week. This does not work for everyone, but for her, she became more comfortable with her *self* and with her clothing choices.

Another patient told me that she was researching plastic surgery because her eye lids "sagged." "I hate my eyes," she protested. She had a pleasant face with nice eyes, and I could not see any flaw with them, and I had a hard time believing that anyone would see a problem with her eyes, but reassurance was not the answer, because her "flaw" was perceived, and it did not matter what others told her as long as she perceived the flaw.

She took some time off from therapy and came back after six weeks. "I had the surgery," she told me. I could not tell at all, and I could see no difference in her. "*I think that you are right. It was always in my head, and it cost a lot of money. But maybe what I need to do is accept that I perceive myself differently from how others do."* And it was this initial act of acceptance, this first step in self-compassion, that led to her ultimate recovery. At first, I had noticed feeling angry at a plastic surgeon who would take a person's money to make unnecessary changes, but then realized that had she not gone through the procedure, she might never have learned to accept herself.

In summary, people with EDs, poor body image, or BDD often experience significant struggles due to self-hatred. When these conditions co-occur with BPD, the self-loathing can be particularly difficult to treat. The origin of self-loathing can vary; in BPD, it often stems from early childhood invalidation and mistreatment, while in EDs, it can arise from significant body dissatisfaction. Additionally, a person with these comorbid conditions may have experienced both early invalidation and maltreatment, as well as profound body dissatisfaction. This means that treatment approaches may need to differ with elements of different approaches added to the therapy, and the concept of self has to be one of the central issues of treatment.

If you are struggling with all of these diagnoses, it might feel as if having to address self-hatred when you have BPD, an eating disorder, BDD, poor body image, and so on, can feel like just one more thing. Interestingly, the more you can find compassion toward yourself, the more likely that these other diagnoses will lose their grip on your life.

Obsessive Compulsive Disorder (OCD)

Obsessive compulsive disorder (OCD) is a mental health disorder that causes people to experience recurring, intrusive, unwanted thoughts, images, or urges. These are called obsessions. They also have repetitive behaviors known as compulsions. These obsessions and compulsions are time consuming and cause significant distress or interfere with daily life. Research has found support for the relationship between OCD and fear of one's self. In a study that looked at the association between OCD and the perception of incompetence in self-domains (the way a person sees themselves in different contexts), (Doron et al. 2008), the researchers found that people with OCD were more prone to draw a negative conclusion about themselves. If the domain of morality was important to them, they tended to consider themselves to be more "immoral, wicked, and crazy on the basis of their unwanted thoughts" as compared to people without OCD.

In short, random unwanted thoughts, which we all experience, are often interpreted by people with OCD as evidence that they may be flawed or even dangerous. The researchers proposed the following idea: When a person with OCD does not think that they are a good or moral person, they become hypervigilant, and then look for clues in their environment that support their self-construct as immoral. When the person becomes hypervigilant, they start to get "immoral" thoughts such as wanting to do others harm. (To be clear, these thoughts in people with OCD are unwanted and intrusive.) When this happens, they conclude that because they have such thoughts, they must be a bad or unethical person. "I am having these thoughts because I must have wanted to harm the other person." They internalize the idea and conclude that they are bad, and the cycle then repeats.

As a patient with OCD told me: *"I have an illogical, internalized, certain, and subjective idea of who I am, and that is that I am a bad, immoral human being. This is based on zero objective facts, and yet these illogical thoughts tell me I am a bad person, and they outweigh the logical and objective idea that I am compassionate and help others."*

Although people with OCD can believe that they are not good people, when I ask them about self-hatred, they don't typically endorse it, as one patient told me: *"No, I don't hate myself. The thoughts are terrible, but I know it's my OCD. If I hate anything, I hate the OCD thoughts that tell me these things."*

Although people with OCD can think of themselves as "bad," I have not found research that people with OCD have higher rates of self-hatred. Typically, if the thought "I hate myself" does arise, it is seen as intrusive and unwanted, which is different from those with core self-loathing who experience the self-hatred as intrinsic and unavoidable.

Depression

SELF-LOATHING IS NOT DEPRESSION: Some mental health professionals tell me that when I discuss core self-hatred, that I am talking about depression, but self-loathing and depression are very different experiences. Most people with depression do NOT hate themselves, and self-loathing is not a criterion of major depressive disorder.

Here is a review of the symptoms necessary to diagnose a person with major depressive disorder, more commonly referred to as depression. According to the DSM (American Psychiatric Association 2022), a person has to experience five or more of the following symptoms. The symptoms have to have been present during the same two-week period and represent a change from previous functioning. Further, that at least one of the symptoms is either (i) a depressed mood or (ii) a loss of interest or pleasure.

1. Depressed mood most of the day, nearly every day, as indicated by either subjective report (e.g., feels sad, empty, hopeless) or observations made by others (e.g., appears tearful).

2. Markedly diminished interest or pleasure in all, or almost all, activities most of the day, nearly every day (as indicated by either subjective account or observation).
3. Significant weight loss when not dieting or weight gain (e.g., a change of more than 5% of body weight in a month) or decrease or increase in appetite nearly every day.
4. Insomnia or hypersomnia nearly every day.
5. Psychomotor agitation or retardation nearly every day (observable by others, not merely subjective feelings of restlessness or being slowed down).
6. Fatigue or loss of energy nearly every day.
7. Feelings of worthlessness or excessive or inappropriate guilt (which may be delusional) nearly every day (not merely self-reproach or guilt about being sick).
8. Diminished ability to think or concentrate, or indecisiveness, nearly every day (either by their subjective account or as observed by others).
9. Recurrent thoughts of death (not just fear of dying), recurrent suicidal ideation without a specific plan, or a suicide attempt or a specific plan for committing suicide.

The one symptom that might be associated with self-hatred is criterion 7: Feelings of worthlessness or excessive or inappropriate guilt nearly every day. What is different with self-hatred versus depression however, is that when the criterion of depression is treated, all of the previous symptoms tend to resolve.

Of my patients who experience self-hatred, some have been diagnosed with depression and some have not. Of the ones who had depression, when the depression was successfully treated, the worthlessness feeling lifted, but the self-loathing did not. It is true that many people with self-loathing also feel worthless and hopeless, but most do not meet clinical criteria for major depression, and even in the cases when they do and the depression is treated, the self-loathing does not respond to the treatment of depression. Medication does not treat self-loathing.

I asked a patient with BPD to differentiate between her experience of self-hatred and depression versus self-hatred and BPD. I asked, "You've experienced self-hatred and depression for a long time. Reflect on self-hatred in depressive episodes versus core self-hatred related to your BPD." This was her answer:

> *"It took a long time for me to be diagnosed with both BPD and depression, partially due to the overlap in some symptoms, and so it was hard to tease out. One of the main symptoms that I have found present in both illnesses is self-hatred. The self-hatred I feel during depressive episodes is very different than the self-hatred I feel from BPD. One of the most obvious differences is that the depression-related self-hatred is episodic and presents only during mood episodes, whereas the BPD self-hatred is continuous. Depression self-hatred is also modifiable, whereas the BPD self-hatred can be coped with, but at my current point in life has not been modifiable. The same coping skills, mostly pulled from DBT, that I use to help alleviate depression self-hatred only help with avoiding or tolerating BPD self-hatred. BPD self-hatred is incredibly insidious. It sits in the background and can be seemingly suppressed for long periods of time while it secretly manipulates you and ruins your life by quietly affecting your sense of identity. Depression self-hatred exists as a symptom. When I feel depression self-hatred, I feel like it is something that I am experiencing, rather than something that is me. When I strip everything down and go down to the core of my identity and self-concept, that is where the BPD self-hatred lives. I have lived through and overcome depression self-hatred during multiple episodes and have come out stronger for it. The BPD self-hatred is something that I don't feel like I could live without. It is who I am and who I will be, and I don't think I will ever be able to escape it."*

This is one of the most articulate reflections on the distinction between core and mood-related, episodic self-hatred, and the impact and experience is clearly stated.

In the next chapter I'll review other personality traits associated with self-hatred. While depression-related self-hatred is episodic and can improve with treatment, core and enduring self-hatred is continuous and deeply ingrained, profoundly affecting how you see yourself. This distinction is crucial for understanding and treating these conditions. Recognizing and addressing the unique characteristics of self-hatred in different contexts is essential for providing comprehensive and effective mental health care.

Chapter 10

Other Personality Traits and Self-Hatred

In this section of the book, I review other topics or published studies where the issue of self-hatred is discussed. I include this chapter for the sake of completeness, however there is not much research on the topics I review. When the following topics are brought up in clinical practice, they are coupled with talk of self-hatred. As with other diagnoses chapters, this one is not intended to be one to self-diagnose. If you identify with some of the ideas in this section, it is important that you consult with a mental health expert.

Narcissism and Self Loathing

> "When I look at narcissism through the vulnerability lens, I see the shame-based fear of being ordinary. I see the fear of never feeling extraordinary enough to be noticed, to be lovable, to belong, or to cultivate a sense of purpose."
>
> —Brené Brown

In Greek mythology, the hunter Narcissus is known for his unsurpassed beauty and in the myth, he rejects all romantic advances. One day he sees his reflection in a pool of water, falls in love with the image, but then tragically, not realizing that the reflection is Narcissus himself, is seduced by the image, falls into the pool of water, and drowns.

In psychology, narcissistic personality disorder is a mental health condition where a person has an unreasonably high sense of their own importance, wants to be seen, and wants people to admire them. They put themselves at the center of all their social interactions. When it comes to the clinical presentation, they present as having toxic levels of self-love. This means that they appear to love themselves to the exclusion of others and in this context, put themselves above everyone else. They are people who tend to name-drop, brag about themselves and their capabilities, and profess their brilliance, and typically tend to be off-putting to those around them.

So why add a section on narcissistic self-love to this book? It seems that, unlike the mythical Narcissus who stared into, and then drowned in, the pool, many narcissists aren't actually in love with themselves. In fact, it could be quite the opposite. New research (Kowalchyk et al. 2021) appears to challenge the idea of the self-loving narcissist. In their research of 270 people with narcissism, (40% male, 60% female), the authors concluded that "narcissism is better understood as a compensatory adaptation to overcome and cover up negative self-worth, instead of genuine grandiosity and grandeur." The authors made a more nuanced distinction between people who have psychopathic traits who "tend to genuinely believe in their own grandiosity and do not present with any hint of insecurities" versus those with vulnerable narcissism who present with significant insecurities and self-loathing and use self-elevating behavior as a compensatory mechanism or defense.

In clinical practice, it's important for clinicians to differentiate between "grandiose narcissism" and "vulnerable narcissism." Grandiose narcissism is often characterized by behaviors that align more closely with psychopathy, including a lack of empathy, compassion, and an inflated sense of self-importance. In contrast, vulnerable narcissism involves individuals who seek reassurance and positive attention rather than power or dominance. These individuals work hard to elevate themselves because they feel deeply inferior. Understanding this distinction is crucial for providing appropriate and effective treatment strategies.

The problem is that in many cases the need for constant external approval from others eventually backfires. At first, it may be the case that others give the person the approval and admiration they want but eventually others are put off by these demands and end up liking the person less and less. And then, when the person with vulnerable narcissism feels less admired, they have to fight even more to get the praise of others. It becomes a vicious cycle of seeking/demanding external praise in order to overcome the self-loathing they feel at a fundamental level. Ironically, in the long run, the person with narcissism isn't rewarded by the demand for admiration. However, because praise works intermittently, they continue to crave external admiration anyway. External validation is never the path to self-compassion. Self-compassion has to come from within.

If you have been diagnosed with narcissism and yet the concept of self-hatred resonates with you, it is possible that some of the ideas in this book may be beneficial. Targeting the deep-seated insecurities, rather than challenging the narcissism itself, will likely be a more beneficial therapeutic approach.

Perfectionism and Self-Hatred

Perfectionism might seem like another odd topic to appear in a book on self-hatred and yet some people with perfectionism recognize the experience of self-hatred. For many people who present for treatment, perfectionism is a painful symptom because it interferes with the satisfaction of day-to-day activities. Typically, people with perfectionism are never satisfied with having done anything well enough. Imagine going throughout the day constantly dissatisfied and upset about how "not perfectly" you did things. For a perfectionist, doing things just right can become both an obsession and a compulsion, and some people with perfectionism meet criteria for obsessive compulsive disorder (OCD) – a review of OCD is beyond the scope and aims of this book.

People with perfectionism can get so caught up in doing things perfectly that they experience an almost unprecedented level of anxiety, and typically this is about how others will judge them. In the context of thinking of their work as imperfect, they begin to anticipate humiliation and shame, and ironically, this can sometimes lead to things not getting done at all. *"If I wasn't sure that I would get a 100% on my essay assignments, I never handed them in. I wrote them but just did not hand them in. I'd rather have an incomplete on my transcript than have my professor think that I was stupid or average,"* is what a junior in college struggling with perfectionism told me. He entered a cycle where he fell further and further behind, even though he had done most of the work! He just didn't hand it in. *"It's like not only will my professor think that I am stupid, but that they will reject me altogether. I just can't stand the thought of it. I spend hours working and reworking each paragraph, each sentence, each word."* This underscores the experience of many people with perfectionism who struggle in interpersonal relationships because the thought of any kind of criticism or rejection is intolerable.

At the same time, the thought of getting close to anyone is also frightening because they fear that their perceived flaws and imperfections will be exposed. In a study (Rozental et al. 2022) of more than 700 students who struggled with procrastination, the researchers found that when perfectionism was the cause of the procrastination, there was a very strong correlation between emotional perfectionism (concerns about making mistakes and not living up to certain standards) and procrastination. The problem with emotional perfectionism is that it is linked to thoughts associated with self-criticism (which we have reviewed elsewhere in the book). These include thoughts like: "I should not feel sad/afraid/inadequate," or "I can't let people know when I am struggling, they will think that I am crazy and weak," or "I need to be happy and positive all the time, so that I don't upset the people around me, and so that I can be the source of comfort for others." All of these statements are self-invalidating and are ultimately impossible to live up to and so the person with perfectionism, unable to live up to an impossible standard, can start to see this as a flaw, and when this is severe enough, self-hatred can begin to set in.

People Pleasing and Self-Hatred

> "You wouldn't worry so much about what others think of you if you realized how seldom they do."
>
> —Eleanor Roosevelt

People pleasing is a behavior that embodies elements of both vulnerable narcissism and perfectionism. It reflects the desire for reassurance and positive attention, characteristics of vulnerable narcissism, with the high standards and fear of failure seen in perfectionism. If you are a people pleaser, you learned it in childhood when you or other people set unrealistic standards and expectations and the need to make other people happy became more important than being authentic and true to yourself. Because these standards and expectations are so impossible to meet on a persistent basis, you might start to judge yourself for being unable to make the other person happy and try even harder, but when you perceive their dissatisfaction, you start to hate yourself.

People pleasers tend to be extremely sensitive and hyper-observant of the reactions of others, perceiving any negative expression as dissatisfaction or criticism. They then tend to change their behavior in order to elicit a positive reaction from the other.

People pleasing is shaped by a combination of intermittent positive and negative reinforcement. The positive reinforcement happens when they see that they are making others happy, and so continue to do all that they can to please others in order to receive the praise of others. On the other hand, negative reinforcement happens – remember that negative reinforcement is the increase in behavior that occurs when an unwanted experience is removed – when they find any perceived or actual criticism so aversive that they try even harder to please the other person, in order to avoid the perceived rejection or dissatisfaction.

In a study (Otani et al. 2018) that compared the difference in core beliefs about self and others in more than 300 healthy volunteers, the researchers found that there was a significant correlation between "sociotropy" scores – where sociotropy refers to people-pleasing behaviors – and negative-self scores. They concluded that these negative core self-beliefs where at the heart of people-pleasing behavior and suggested that these core beliefs were also implicated in becoming people pleasing. The researchers gave the following example, an experience that many readers of this book will identify with: "I am unloved" gives rise to the self-construct: "It is important to be liked and approved by others," and in this context they embark in the unrelenting pursuit of others' approval as a way of dismissing the unlovable self.

EXERCISE 1

Am I a people pleaser?

I am overly apologetic: Y/N

I take responsibility for other people's feelings: Y/N

I tend to agree with people and say yes, even when I don't agree, in order to avoid conflict: Y/N

EXERCISE 2

Overcoming People Pleasing

Identify Your Values: Take time to clearly define your core values. Reflect on what matters most to you and what you want to live by.

Practice Setting Boundaries: When faced with requests or situations that conflict with your values, practice saying no. Be proud to stick to your values by saying no and maintaining your integrity.

Manage Guilt: If you feel guilty after saying no, revisit your values. Reflect on why sticking to your values is important.

Assess Your Progress: Regularly check in on your behavior to see if you are continuing to people please. If you find that you are still struggling with people-pleasing behaviors, consider professional help to help you overcome these challenges.

Bullying Behavior and Self-Hatred

Research has shown that children who were abused are much more likely to become bullies at school. In one paper (Ma 2023) that included various forms of bullying – physical bullying, verbal bullying, relational bullying, and cyber bullying, the authors wanted to confirm previous research that abuse predicted school bullying, and then further they hypothesized that self-hatred was a factor in the bullying.

The authors shared the following reflections on self-hatred: "It is a long-term or repeated aversion to certain aspects of the self, resulting in a series of negative avoidance and rejection reactions," as well as a "negative self-conscious emotion, a negative and unclear part of the self-concept." They recognized that childhood abuse distorted a child's sense of themselves, and that this was in part because they believed that they had caused the abuse, felt guilty that they had done so, could not let go of the guilt, and because of this they then hate themselves. Their research included 587 students (262 boys and 325 girls), of which 358 were middle schoolers and 229 high school students.

They found that the effect of childhood abuse on self-loathing was significant. Not surprisingly, the more a child experienced abuse, the higher their level of self-hatred. However, in the study, self-loathing alone did not predict bullying behavior.

The researchers considered that if child abuse was "justified" by the abuser, meaning that the abuser explained to the child why they had abused them, that the child would internalize that it is OK to hurt others by justifying it. However, if instead, the child internalized the belief that they were abused because they were "bad" leading to self-hatred, that this experience would not predict bullying.

What this means is that many bullies have been abused as children, but not all abused children are bullies. Children who are abused who hear justifications from their abuser as to why the abuse is "justified" are more likely to be bullies and use justification for bullying others. Abused children who end up believing that they are bad are much more likely to end up hating themselves.

Moving Forward: Addressing Self-Hatred

For the first 10 chapters, you have been reading about the nature of self-hatred, how it develops, and the lived experience. I hope that by now, what you have read will have convinced you that you were not at fault for the things that happened to you, that the things that happened to you taught you to hate yourself and that what you learned you can unlearn. Next, we'll review the approaches that have been considered to target self-hatred, those that have worked, those that have not helped, and those that hold some promise.

Part 4

Treatment and Overcoming Barriers to Treatment

Chapter 11

Targeting Self-Hatred

> "The way you think about yourself determines your reality. You are not being hurt by the way people think about you. Many of those people are a reflection of how you think about yourself."
>
> —Shannon L. Alder

Although there are therapies that treat the symptoms of anorexia, obsessive compulsive disorder (OCD), post traumatic stress disorder (PTSD), and other conditions, there is no therapy that focuses specifically on self-hatred. In Chapter 14, you will see what those with lived experience say about what helped them. Even though the therapies and approaches I review in this chapter don't have an evidence base for targeting self-hatred, they are the ones that I am trained in and have the potential to reduce the experience of self-loathing. Having a broad understanding of these therapies will lay the groundwork for the exercises in Chapter 14.

Even though I cover the major therapy types, this is not a book on types of therapy. The review of these therapies is so that you have an understanding of what they are. I don't include too many exercises in this chapter, although there are some when the topic is directly tied to self-hatred, or reflecting on the topic might help you shift the core belief. I don't go extensively into each type nor offer the multitude of techniques that each teaches. If any of them is of interest to you, there are online resources where you can find therapists who practice these therapies.

Addressing Core Beliefs

> "The internal war you wage with yourself may not be seen by others but is always felt by you!"
>
> —Lorraine Nilon

Core beliefs are strong, long-term beliefs that we all have and that help us understand who we are and how the world works. These beliefs begin to form in our early childhood and influence our personality, our behaviors, the decisions we make as well as our mental health. In some ways they act as rules as to how to interact with others and the world and dictate the behavior that we will accept and tolerate. They are shaped by our families, our culture, our faith, and our experiences.

1. **Universal Norms or Ethical Values:** These are widely accepted and agreed upon by society at large.

   Most core beliefs are ones that many others in society agree with; for example, I believe that:

   Murder is wrong.

   We should be kind to others.

   We shouldn't steal.

2. **Common Practical Beliefs or Social Norms:** These beliefs are sensible and widely shared, reflecting everyday responsibilities and norms.

   There are other beliefs that make a lot of sense at the individual level, but are shared by many others; such as, I believe that:

   I should brush my teeth regularly.

   I should show up to work on time.

   I should obey the speed limit.

   Relationships need effective communication.

3. **Personal Core Beliefs:** These beliefs are deeply personal and may or may not be shared by others.

There are yet other beliefs that are much more personal and may or might not be shared by others, but are true to you; such as, I believe that:

I am trustworthy.

I am dependable.

I am loveable.

4. **Harmful Core Beliefs:** These beliefs cause significant distress and can be damaging to one's well-being.

   And then there are core beliefs that cause distress and damage to the self; such as, I believe that:

   I don't belong.

   People are out to get me.

   Everyone is selfish.

   I'll never be good enough for someone else.

EXERCISE

Before reading on, start with reflecting on your general and specific core beliefs.

ANSWER: My core beliefs are:

____

____

____

____

REFLECTION: Once you have considered your core beliefs, think about the circumstances and experiences that led you to develop your core beliefs.

Core beliefs and depression: There is a theory of how depression develops known as the cognitive model of depression. It was developed by Dr. Aaron Beck, a preeminent researcher and clinician in the field of cognitive psychology (1987). He theorized that depressive symptoms were generated and maintained by a combination of maladaptive cognitions, and, according to the cognitive model, people with depression are prone to focus on negative thoughts and experiences, perceive life events as more negative, ruminate about negative thoughts, recall the negative aspects of situations more than the positive ones, and then have negative views of who they are as people. It makes a lot of sense that if you experienced life in this way, that you would be depressed.

His theory also resonates for people with anxiety, for instance if you have anxiety and have a core belief that you won't be able to handle negative experiences, a core belief that might sound like: "I'm a weak person," or "everything I do goes wrong," you are less likely to try new things and more likely to be nervous in novel situations.

And so, if core beliefs are central to anxiety and depression, can they be changed? Recall that these are typically persistent and deep-rooted and yet for many of these, research has shown that although it can be challenging, once you identify them, with patience, practice, and self-compassion they do begin to change. You have to acknowledge that it exists and then name it. That is the first step in changing it. The next step is to review the ways in which the core belief is impacting your life, and even imagine what your life would look like if you didn't have that belief. For example, let's say you've become aware that you firmly believe it's not possible to work a night shift at a hospital and have a healthy relationship at home. This core belief may be keeping you from applying for a job that may be ideal for you, that you have trained for, and that you are skilled at. If you didn't have this core belief, you could apply for that nursing job while confirming that you have a supportive and loving partner at home.

Is Self-Hatred a Core Belief?

In the strictest sense of the definition, yes. However, different from the previous example, for people with self-loathing, they do not see self-hatred as a core belief. They see it as a part of who they are, and so even though they might be open to the idea that they can do difficult work in therapy, they don't believe that they can do anything about self-hatred.

A patient once quipped: *"Didn't Freud say that: 'sometimes a piece of shit is just a piece of shit?'"*

I must admit I chuckled at that. Many of the people I work and have worked with for such a long time are deeply thoughtful, likeable, and funny.

Another patient who was new to our treatment was referred to me because of self-hatred. I asked her to think about her past self and whether she hated the little girl she had been. I asked her if her conclusion of self-hatred was immutable. These are her reflections:

> *"I was asked to consider the mere possibility that I could be wrong. That the dialog that I have so tirelessly maintained could be flawed. Flawed in both reasoning and within the premise itself. I was asked to look at the little girl that I used to be. She looked in the mirror and drowned in the longing to cut her stomach off with scissors. Would I give her those scissors today? No, of course not. But today, do I drown in the same desperate desire? Yes, and if it were a rational possibility, I would act on it as well.*
>
> *"How is it that we are always changing yet the dialog I created so long ago seems to remain constant? How is it possible that the little girl that I once was already carried the weight of unavoidable shame from a guilt that had yet to be discovered.*
>
> *"No harm no foul right? Apparently not.*
>
> *"Where was the harm? Was it the mere fact of my existence? But looking at that little girl, how could I say that? I don't hate her today so why did I hate her then? However, I deeply hate myself now. In 20 years when I look back at pictures of myself now will I feel the same as I do looking at 5-year-old me? If in 20 years I look back and ask myself 'how could you hate that young woman?' then what the fuck is the point and why am I so stuck in this dialog that is increasingly seeming less logical?*
>
> *"My dialog of self-hatred was unknowingly created and unwillingly strengthened through years of invalidation, inflicted pain, and outright assault. The issue is that no matter how this dialog came to be, I have knowingly been maintaining it with*

every fiber within myself. Every thought, followed by many feelings, and far too many behaviors, have acted as evidence to help the loathing grow.

"Hate is a strong word. But it doesn't come close to describing how I have grown to feel about myself. The dialog that was created, maintained, and strengthened is more harmful than anything I have ever known. The pain is insufferable.

"Yet here I am. I still hate myself. And I hate myself so much that it's hard for me to believe that I shouldn't hate myself. Will I still hate me in the future?

"I ask you in return. 'If it is core to me, how can that possibly change?'"

What Does Not Work

> "In the midst of my pain of heart and frantic effort of principle, I abhorred myself. I had no solace from self-approbation: none even from self-respect. I had injured—wounded—left my master. I was hateful in my own eyes."
>
> —From *Jane Eyre* by Charlotte Brontë

In this quote, Jane is expressing her feelings of self-loathing and internal conflict after leaving Mr. Rochester, her employer and the man she loves, after realizing he is married. Jane struggles with the pain of her decision and feels deep regret and self-hatred for leaving Rochester, despite knowing it was the morally right choice. The path away from self-hate is not simple. Simply saying approving things about herself is not enough to reduce Jane Eyre's self-hatred. But if being nice to yourself does not work, then what?

The heading "What Does Not Work" is a bit misleading because some of the ideas that will work come from the approaches listed that follow. The issue lies in how these therapies are applied. The problem is none of the therapies explicitly treat self-hatred, so there are no specific practices or protocols offered to treat self-hatred. In fact, if used without considering the broader picture of self-loathing, these therapies may make you feel invalidated and, in some cases, may make you experience more self-hatred. This is because even when you apply the recommendations to your life, even if they change other aspects of your life, they don't change the self-hatred. Then it can feel that this "proves" that nothing will help.

One reason for this is what we've discussed earlier in this book – many therapists do not recognize self-loathing as its own entity but rather as a symptom of some other diagnosis, and imagine that if the disorder is treated, say depression or PTSD, that self-hatred will lift. However, this strategy is not always effective for self-hatred and may even work in reverse, leading to increased feelings of inadequacy and self-loathing. If a therapist suggests that a therapy will help, and it does not, you might conclude that you are even more defective than you thought, and then experience even more self-hatred.

I once suggested to a patient that only he could change his self-hatred, meaning that I could give him certain tools and ideas to practice, but that only he himself could do the work and make the changes necessary to change any negative belief of core self. I told him that he had to do the work, and that it had to start with challenging the certainty of self-hatred.

He came back to session the next week and said: *"Yeah, you might be right, and maybe it's true, but here's the issue: I hate myself so deeply and think that I am such a shitty disgusting person that I wouldn't want to 'like' this me. This is why I am constantly trying to change myself to become someone I deem worth accepting or even liking. But look where trying to change got me. I was overweight so I got neck deep in anorexia. Yup, no luck there. So, turns out I am in fact stuck with myself for the rest of my life. So, I understand that it is on me to stop hating myself, but the idea of accepting myself as I am now, is my worst fear. I am so repulsed by myself but simultaneously believe that that is the correct way to feel about myself because of how much I hate myself. That's the irony. Hating myself is the one thing I'm doing right. So how am I supposed to stop doing the one thing I am doing right and all of the sudden just decide it's time to try liking myself? Just doesn't seem like a viable option ... so am I just kind of fucked?"*

This concept resonates so much with people who experience self-hatred. Over the year of doing research into this book, my wonderful patient collaborators have shared what does work and what does not work in tackling self-loathing.

EXERCISE

Have you ever tried to tackle self-hatred? Have therapists suggested ideas to address your self-hatred? What has your experience been? Have any of the ideas worked? And if so, which ones? Which ideas have not worked?

ANSWER:

____

____

____

____

____

____

____

Psychotherapy Approaches

In practice, there are two main approaches using traditional therapies to target self-hatred. These are acceptance-focused and change-focused therapies. Acceptance-focused strategies are ones that are validating, compassionate, and deeply recognize the suffering of the person. You can imagine a kind, attentive therapist who accepts you for who you are and validates your experiences, including those of self-hatred. Patients' experiences of such therapies often leave them feeling deeply understood on the one hand, but on the other hand leave them feeling stuck in self-hatred and with a persistent lack of self-worth, wondering to themselves: "I have a great therapist who cares about me, but I still hate myself. How do I change that?" Simply being listened to, cared for, and understood, is not a solution to overcoming self-hatred.

Change-focused strategies tend to point out the flaws in a person's thinking and behavior and recommend strategies to change the way a person thinks or acts; however, for people with self-hatred these strategies often leave patients feeling invalidated because techniques such as the recommendation that the person practice loving self-compassion makes the patient feel that they haven't been listened to, "You are asking me to do the impossible" or, "Oh you think it's that easy? You're telling me that all I have to do to overcome how much I hate myself is tell myself how much I love myself?"

One patient told me: *"You asked me to think about this, and it seemed absurd at first, but here are my reflections: It has been difficult for me to even think of practicing self-compassion or self-love because I feel undeserving of it. I feel like a horrible person for even considering it as something I'm allowed to do because I feel that makes me egotistical and conceited in a manner that causes harm to others. Self-compassion and self-love also feel impossible for me to practice because it runs so counter to my internal dialogue that I cannot internalize positive messaging toward myself. If I had to choose between self-compassion and self-love, I would pursue self-compassion because that feels more realistic and aligns with my values."*

Her writing expresses the challenge so clearly.

Dr. Roy Krawitz (2012) theorized that the well-meaning encouragement from clinicians such as trying to get their patients to work on cultivating positive self-esteem often backfired and left their patients feeling even more self-hatred thoughts. This is because therapists can make it sound so easy to do, but then when the patient finds it nearly impossible, they feel that this highlights just how flawed they are, and then experience even more self-hatred.

Psychodynamic and more relationally based therapies would attempt to address self-hatred through the generation of insight into the early problems with their caregivers, the ones that led to a distorted and self-deprecating self-image. The problem with these approaches is that you can't go back and correct what was done, and many people then spend a lot of thought time ruminating on how they were mistreated and then end up hating themselves more, feeling that it must have been because of how flawed they were. The question is less, "what can my therapist do," but more "what can I do?" Ultimately, the power is in your hands to change self-hatred.

A relational therapist might be able to point out the pattern of maltreatment, but it takes your hard work to recognize that it led to a belief about yourself that is false.

Before considering ideas that do work, here is what the limited research says on tackling self-hatred. Although there is no research that the abovementioned approaches have helped, because any approach to targeting self-loathing is derived from these therapies, it is important for you to understand them and what the literature says about them.

Self-Compassion

> "Genuine self-love is the most profound experience in the universe. However, it usually takes time, sincere dedication, and discipline to develop. We are surrounded by so many images, beliefs, and behaviors that reinforce the idea of self-hatred every day that it can be extremely difficult for us to connect to the love inside of us."
>
> —Mateo Sol

In many ways, focusing on self-compassion seems like the most obvious way to tackle self-loathing. After all, if you hate yourself, it stands to reason that you should practice loving yourself. What research shows about the practice of self-compassion is that it helps reduce the symptoms of depression. Typically, this form of self-compassion is done by performing caring behaviors toward the self, as well as expressing and communicating feelings of warmth and safety toward the self. Several studies have also explored the relationship between self-compassion and well-being. People with high self-compassion have fewer psychiatric symptoms, more overall well-being, and a better quality of life (Neff et al. 2007; Neely et al. 2009; Van Dam et al. 2011).

It is important to underscore what you read earlier in the book: self-hatred and depression are not the same. While they can coexist, they are distinct experiences that typically require different approaches, although many of the approaches will have common concepts. Depression often involves a pervasive sense of sadness, loss of interest, and lack of energy, which can be alleviated through cognitive behavioral therapy and medication. On the other hand, self-hatred is characterized by a profound and persistent negative self-view that is more resistant to simple acts of self-care and compassion, and does not yield at all to medication. While it is ideal to have a nurturing and compassionate self-stance, addressing self-hatred requires a deeper exploration of the cognitive and emotional roots of this negative self-perception, and treatments must be tailored to challenge and transform these core beliefs.

Treatment developers have created a handful of compassion-focused therapies (CFTs) that you'll read about shortly. For people with enduring core self-hatred, none of them have worked, at least not in the patients I have worked with. In fact, many have told me that if I prescribe self-compassion exercises, that they won't do them. *"Have you heard the people on podcasts who try to get you to practice. Firstly, their voice turns me off. It's so sweet and soft and 'ooh love yourself and invite kindness into your heart' and all that bullsh!t. I mean seriously, hearing some of their voices makes me hate myself more because I can't imagine that anyone has lived such a wonderful life that they can talk that way. I hate therapist voices, you know the ones that don't sound natural, and they only use in the office and would never speak to another human being that way! And no, don't ask me how that makes me feel,"* warned one skeptical patient who was ready to tackle her skepticism. Nevertheless, my task is to get you to care for yourself at least a little before you care for yourself a lot, and because of this, these therapies are worth reviewing. So, even **though none of the following approaches have been shown to reduce self-hatred, it is in large part because none have been studied for self-hatred, and certainly self-hatred should be a focus of these approaches.**

There are three major therapies that consider self-compassion in their approach. I discuss dialectical behavior therapy (DBT) separately:

a. CFT is a form of therapy developed for people whose mental health conditions are linked to high shame and self-criticism. It aims to help people respond to self-criticism with self-kindness and compassion. In a review (Leaviss and Uttley 2015) of 14 articles on CFT, the authors concluded: "The findings from the included studies were, in the most part, favorable to CFT, and in particular seemed to be effective for people who were high in self-criticism." (See section on self-criticism in Chapter 3.) Nevertheless, the authors recognized that the quality of the trials was not great, and that CFT seemed to work best with mood disorders, such as depression. I found no studies using CFT for self-hatred.

b. Acceptance and commitment therapy (ACT) is a therapy that focuses on helping people to stop avoiding, denying, and struggling with their inner emotions and, instead, accept that these deeper feelings are present, and that even if the feelings are negative, that negative feelings are not a reason why a person should not succeed and move forward in their lives. In ACT, people focus on accepting the hardships in their lives and commit to make the changes necessary to change behavior that keeps them stuck. ACT uses mindfulness, including compassion mindfulness, as well as acceptance skills to address the obstacles that get in the way of what matters to the person. However, as with CFT, there is no research on the use of ACT for self-hatred.

c. Mindfulness-based cognitive therapy (MBCT) is a modified form of cognitive therapy (see following section) that incorporates mindfulness practices, meditation, and breathing exercises. It was developed to address depression and teaches patients to be in the here and now rather than ruminating on a painful past. It teaches them how to identify, and break away from, negative thought patterns that can lead to depression. In recent modifications, it explicitly makes the promotion of self-compassion an aim of therapy and highlights the improvement in self-compassion as a mechanism of change especially in people with depression. And again, there are no studies that show that MBCT reduces self-hatred.

I asked some patients about whether they had ever heard of the practice of self-compassion and if they had considered it. Here are some of their answers:

Answer 1: "*Yes, I have tried many times. I have been in and out of treatment places since I was 13. I have been to facilities 15 different times. I tried so hard to tell myself positive things and that I love myself but that felt so unearthly. They say fake it until you make it, and I sure did fake it. I just never could make it. This is until I learned DBT and really leaned into it. I have known the skills since I first got hospitalized at the age of 13. I honestly thought they were dumb and unhelpful. But as I tried them at least, I learned I could change, and this was just a language I could replace with another. This is hard though and I not only have to learn a new language, but I am going to do trauma work to help with that.*"

Answer 2: "*I've thought about it but it doesn't work and it feels very pointless. It never works because I'm too good at convincing myself that I deserve to hate myself or be hated. It feels impossible to believe good things about myself. Self-compassion never sticks.*"

Answer 3: "*Did I ever think of it? No. Did my previous therapist? Yes. He was all about self-affirmations. I tried putting post-its up in my room with positive affirmations. I'm trying to come up with a way to explain this that will really drive the point home, but I don't think I can. If you simply repeat something to yourself that you know is not true, it will not force your brain to believe it. No matter how many times you say it. There has to be some part of you that is receptive to the information and willing to entertain it. Neither of those things apply to me. The BIGGEST hang up with practicing self-compassion is believing that you deserve it.*"

"*So that's quite a conundrum, right? How do you convince someone who hates themselves to believe they deserve to love themselves? Nobody was able to figure that out for me. Almost nobody.*"

Answer 4: "*I understand the idea but where does one start? How do you find those small parts to be compassionate toward when self-hatred is so widespread?*"

Answer 5: "*I know you have asked me to practice this for a few months. Honestly, I have not been able to successfully practice self-compassion. I believe it is because my "feeling" of self-hatred is so deep-seated and inherent that I saw it as a truth rather than something that could be challenged, questioned, or even put aside.*"

Answer 6: "*I heard about practicing self-compassion or self-love in outpatient therapy, particularly in DBT. I found the concept laughable and have been very reluctant to try it, in part due to feeling as though it is something that is impossible for me to achieve.*"

Cognitive Behavior Therapy (CBT)

> "Perhaps the most liberating moment in my life was when I realized that my self-loathing was not a product of my inadequacy but, rather, a product of my thoughts."
>
> —Vironika Tugaleva

What is cognitive behavioral therapy (CBT)? Here's a quick overview:

CBT is a form of therapy that has been found to be effective in many psychiatric diagnoses such as depression, anxiety disorders, substance use problems, eating disorders, and many others. It is a powerful intervention, and, in many studies, CBT has been shown to be as effective as, or even more effective than, other forms of psychotherapy or psychiatric medications.

Core Principles of CBT Theory

The theory behind CBT is that psychological problems are:

1. To some degree based on erroneous or unhelpful ways of thinking.
2. In part based on learned patterns of unhelpful behavior.

And then, based on the aforementioned, that:

3. People struggling with these problems can learn more skillful and helpful ways of coping with them, which in turn relieves the problems, and which then leads to more effective functioning in life.

Although CBT treatment also focuses on behavior (the B in CBT), the C in CBT stands for cognitive, meaning thinking, and consequently, CBT treatment tends to focus on getting people to change thinking patterns, by using the following general strategies. They:

a. Learn to recognize the particular distortions in their way of thinking that lead to problems and then learn to reevaluate the thoughts through the lens of reality.

   For example, there is a distortion known as filtering. Filtering is the way that a person ignores all of the positive things in their life to focus solely on the negative. It's a cognitive trap that leads to dwelling on a single negative aspect of a situation and filtering out all the good ones. An example of this was a former patient of mine who had spent many years in and out of hospitals. Eventually, through hard work, she stopped using self-destructive behaviors, stopped the annual practice of being hospitalized every fall, the anniversary of a significant trauma, married her long-term boyfriend, had two wonderful kids, (I know this as she brought her family to meet me!) and went to grad school and eventually became a therapist. Now, in her first semester, she got Bs in two subjects. She had been a straight A student in high school and undergrad, before the years of hospitalization. She called me up, very upset about her "terrible grades," and how they were proof that she should "never have applied to be a therapist," and that she was considering dropping out of school. Her husband told her that she had done well and that it was a relatively minor bump in the road.

Because she was in an emotional state, she interpreted his behavior as trying to placate her, even though she "knew" that he "thought she was stupid." I pointed out how she had fallen into a filtering trap. Rather than zooming out and seeing all that she had accomplished, and further, recognizing that she was a little rusty for having missed so much school, and having young children in her life, she filtered out the immense work that she had done and focused only on the perceived negative.

b. Learn how thoughts, emotions and behaviors are interconnected.

Continuing with the previous example, her thought "I got terrible grades" led to the emotional experience of sadness and despair which then led to the urge to quit school.

c. Gain more insight into the behavior and motivation of others.

My patient was able to step back and recognize her loving husband had always been supportive and how her strong emotions had led her to misinterpret his motivations.

d. Learn, and then use, new adaptive problem-solving skills to cope with difficult situations.

In my patient's case, she knew the thinking traps and skills. She recognized that she had fallen into an automatic thought pattern and was able to use cognitive restructuring, a technique where she recognizes the destructive nature of her thinking, and see what had happened from a more affirming and less destructive point of view.

e. Generalize new skills to everyday situations and in so doing develop a greater sense of confidence in your own capabilities.

My patient was able to take on the challenges of being back at school, as an older student and with a family and be less judgmental of herself in other situations where outcomes weren't perfect.

What Can Help: When Self-Blame Is a Core Part of Your Self-Loathing

If you are someone who tends to blame themselves a lot, here are some useful practices from cognitive behavioral therapy:

- **Decentering through mindful awareness.** This is the ability to stand back and view a thought as a cognitive event: as an opinion, and not necessarily a fact. Your task is to label the process that is present in the thinking, rather than engaging in the content of the thinking. If you are blaming yourself, try saying "I am blaming myself again." You want to catch the behavior of blaming yourself and then label it, rather that engaging with the thought and going down the spiral of negative self-attribution.
- **Reattribution.** This is the practice of identifying the factors that may have contributed to a negative outcome, the ones aside from you. You then consider just how much each of those factors contributed to the outcome. For instance, say that you went to a party, and someone spiked your drink, and you got so sick that you had to go to the hospital. Yes, you went to the party. However, some person put a drug in your drink. You never asked for that, nor wanted it. The person who spiked your drink had a lot of responsibility for what happened, and then the drug also caused you to be sick. The point here is to not blame yourself for absolutely everything that happened, and even if you can take some responsibility, you are making a shift from taking total responsibility to seeing a more balanced view with many other factors.
- **Cognitive restructuring by using thought records.** A thought record is a common exercise used by cognitive behavioral therapists and is a practical way to capture the way you think about a specific situation. Typically, it is a written practice and goes something like this: Say that you invite people for dinner and the restaurant was overbooked. (You should do this practice with a specific and true

experience in your life.) That is the event that prompts what happens next. For instance, you might have the automatic thought such as "I am to blame for everything." Your task then is to reevaluate the thought through considering all of the evidence that your conclusion is true, and then to arrive at different conclusions.

EXERCISE

For example, other than concluding that you are to blame for everything, you might ask yourself:

a. "Are there other explanations for what happened?"

b. "Are there other contributing factors that I may be missing, or that I am downplaying?"

c. "If a neutral observer, understood what was happening, would they say I was totally to blame?"

d. Alternatively, "If the restaurant situation had happened to one of my friends, would I say that they were entirely to blame?"

e. "Can I use non-judgmental and accurate language to describe what happened?"

f. Even if you recognize that you are partly at fault, ask yourself, "What were my intentions? Do I typically intend to inconvenience my friends by having them wait at a full restaurant that has overbooked?"

EXERCISE

Testing your beliefs and assumptions. Do you believe that blaming yourself gives you more control? Or that you want to beat others to the punch, "If I blame myself, people are less likely to blame me." You can always test these ideas out to see if they are accurate. For instance, you could write down: Everyone will blame me if I don't blame myself. Next, see what happens if the next time something negative happens you don't blame yourself. Does everyone come out of the woodwork to blame you? Write down the outcome and see if your expectation, that you will be blamed, is violated or validated.

Does it help? As mentioned earlier, if you are judging your behavior and actions as the reason why something failed, blaming yourself could have the benefit of learning from the experience and then doing something different the next time. "In blaming myself, I won't make the same mistake again, and I will start studying for the exam earlier next time." If, on the other hand, self-blame is used to entrench negative attributes that have no basis in fact or reality, then it is not helpful.

Tackling Self-Contempt

> "Cause I'm not much to want to learn from my mistakes
> I tend to hide behind the habits I should shake
> If you really knew me, I'm not sure you'd like me
> So I'll remain concealed in regret"
>
> —Lyrics from Self Loathing by Days n' Daze

In Chapter 1 we reviewed how self-contempt has some significant differences from, as well as some similarities to, self-loathing. In focusing on self-contempt, researchers (Sallin et al. 2021) examined the role of expressed self-contempt in therapy for patients with borderline personality disorder (BPD). They found two interesting results. The first is that expressed self-contempt did not change during the treatment. Again, we see a failure of therapy to address an experience related to self-loathing. What is more surprising is the disconnect between the perceptions of therapists and their patients; people with high self-contempt rated their therapeutic alliance with their therapists as weak, whereas therapists rated their therapeutic alliance with their patients as strong!

The researchers hypothesized that patients with self-contempt could be less confident in engaging in a therapeutic relationship, with its implied closeness and that this is because of a devaluating self-perception of being inadequate and feeling that they are likely to be rejected. But then how is it that therapists felt that the therapeutic alliance was strong? They hypothesized that when patients expressed self-contempt, that this was interpreted by the therapist as the patient being vulnerable and an indication that the patients trusted the relationship. They also theorized that when patients expressed self-contempt, that this could provoke an empathic reaction in the therapist who might see their patient's harsh and painful self-treatment as a manifestation of their suffering and cause the therapist to feel closer to their patient.

The researchers concluded that their results highlighted the need to better understand self-contempt and to be attentive to its effect on clinical symptomatology and therapeutic relationship during therapy, which is not dissimilar from what my goals for this book are.

Dialectical Behavior Therapy (DBT)

Although I have been trained in the other therapeutic approaches I mention in this book, the one I have been practicing for the past nearly 20 years is DBT. It is derived from CBT and was developed for suicidal people whose suicidal thoughts and behaviors come from the pain of overwhelming emotions and self-deprecating thoughts. DBT was developed by Dr. Marsha Linehan (1993), a psychologist at the University of Washington. Linehan recognized that when emotionally sensitive children were invalidated, meaning that when their private experiences were rejected by others, that they began to invalidate themselves and then see themselves as defective. Before DBT, the traditional forms of therapy were CBT and psychodynamic therapies. Of all the forms of therapy for suicidal people, DBT has the most evidence supporting its use as an approach that reduces suicidality and self-destructiveness.

The word "dialectical" in the context of DBT means that there are different truths to any perspective and that the task is to integrate or synthesize truths, even if these truths seem to be complete opposites.

For example: Many people who have painful emotions find that self-injury through cutting helps to reduce the level of emotional pain. Now if you told someone that you were cutting yourself, most people would say that you have a problem. However, for you cutting is not necessarily a problem. It is a solution to the problem of intense suffering. Cutting is a problem and a solution at the same time. In this situation what an outsider sees as a problem (one truth), is actually seen as a solution (another truth) to the person cutting. How can you synthesize these seemingly opposite ideas? The synthesis is that cutting is an effective short-term solution, yet long-term a maladaptive problem, to the experience of intense and painful emotions. Other, healthier, ways can be used to address the problem of painful emotions although maybe not as immediately effective. Seeing both sides leads to a more complete understanding of the cutting behavior.

Dialectics is about combining opposite ideas into a new idea. Opposites abound in DBT including integrating Eastern acceptance philosophy, derived from Zen, with Western change techniques derived from CBT. The most fundamental of these seemingly opposing truths is that in order to help someone change who they are or how they see themselves, they must first accept the other person, or accept themselves, as they are.

In DBT, change is integrated with acceptance. What DBT has shown is that once a person feels that they are accepted and understood by their therapist, that they are then able to learn the skill and make the changes necessary to deal with the stuff of life that causes suffering.

What type of problems is DBT useful for?

DBT is especially effective for people who have difficulty managing and regulating their emotions. Many people who benefit from DBT recognize that they are emotionally sensitive: If you are a person who tends to feel things deeper than others, quicker than others, and when you have an emotional reaction, tends to take longer to come down to your emotional baseline. If you are looking for a therapy, DBT could be for you. Being emotionally sensitive is not the problem. Instead, problems arise when the behaviors that you engage in are dependent on your mood. Imagine that when you are in a good mood, you can get anything done, but when you are in a bad mood, you can't complete the things that are necessary to get done. For people with emotions that are difficult to control, this means that many necessary activities don't get done, or take a lot longer to get done. This could definitely impact you, but it might impact others as well. Imagine that a pilot could only fly when they were in a good mood, but not in a bad mood. It could make for a dangerous situation if halfway through the flight their mood went from good to bad.

The bottom line is that DBT can provide the tools to help you manage your emotions more effectively, ensuring that your mood does not dictate your ability to function and perform essential tasks.

The concept of inhibited grieving: In DBT there is a focus of treatment where inhibited grieving is targeted. Inhibited grieving includes all the active and passive ways that people use to avoid or escape their thoughts or emotions and in particular the thoughts and emotions relating to grief.

I asked a patient about her self-hatred, and she said: *"I have never wanted to even think about it. It's just there."* When I asked her why she didn't want to explore it, she said. *"I was adopted. Someone discarded me, and then the people who adopted me treated me very badly, especially when they had their own biological child. So, what should I conclude. That my birth mom didn't want me and that my adoptive parents saw me as flawed. I was broken. I am broken. I am the broken child that no one wants. Of course, I hate myself. And you want me to look at all of that?"*

I teared up, she was such a wonderful young person. She needed to examine the grief of rejection, but she felt that it was too painful a task. When life has not been kind, when people have disappointed us, when we feel that we were deprived of the things that others got, most people feel sad. But for some, the sadness can feel so unbearable that we simply don't want to examine it. Instead of grieving the past, some people inhibit that grieving, and this can be particularly true when examining the losses in your life means exposing yourself to comments and relationships that taught you to hate yourself. The most effective way to be sad, is to be sad, to experience the feelings of sorrow as they arise and as they are remembered, to seek support and validation, to engage in the fabric of your life and to be kind to yourself. When engaging in the grief, thoughts and other emotions might arise. You might also experience the regret that you didn't do more to fight for yourself and judge yourself for having been weak at times. These are all common reactions when you target inhibited grieving.

EXERCISE

Think about the things that feel unfair about your childhood. The ways in which you didn't get your needs met. The ways in which you were treated. The things you missed out on.

ANSWER: Write these down and with each answer, write down the emotions that each of these experiences elicited.

____

____

____

____

____

____

____

____

Specific Skills for Suffering

DBT focuses on four specific skill sets. The skills make sense given the problems that bring people into DBT:

Mindfulness: This is the practice of being fully present and aware, and doing so without getting caught up in judgments. The idea of focusing the mind on the present moment is much harder than at first it may seem, but as with most things, the more you practice, the easier it becomes. Mindfulness is the core practice of DBT because many people who come to DBT, spend a lot of their time dwelling in the suffering of past hurts and traumas, or worrying about a future that has not yet happened. They also beat themselves up with negative self-talk. What mindfulness research shows is that through the practice of being present and more aware, dealing with future problems becomes easier. Mindfulness also helps reduce strong emotions and improve or heal damaged relationships, including the damaged relationship with yourself.

Distress tolerance: For people who come to DBT, their emotions and thoughts about themselves can feel unbearable. It's understandable that if you are in severe emotional pain, that you want immediate relief. Unfortunately, in many situations, there aren't many immediate answers, or at least few that are healthy, and this is often when many turn to effective, yet maladaptive, answers. By this I mean that they turn to solutions that actually work, although only in the short term, and then have negative consequences in the long run. Solutions such as drugs, dangerous sexual encounters, or self-injury are effective. Many people don't realize that these solutions do work, but only temporarily. The solutions, however, typically last for only a few minutes and often leave the person feeling worse in the long run. Solutions with such short-lived effects aren't ideal. Imagine that you had to get your appendix removed or your tonsils taken out. Now imagine your surgeon saying, "Your operation was a success. Why don't you come back next week, and I'll take them out again." Sadly, people with chronic self-loathing often engage in behaviors that end up hurting themselves, and further, feel that they deserve the negative consequences of these behaviors.

Because life can present many situations that aren't solvable in the moment, DBT has a module of distress tolerance skills to get you through those moments. The skills teach you to manage stressful moments more effectively, while preserving your self-respect and dignity. The idea is to get you through the moment until you can apply other, longer-lasting, skills, or solve the problem altogether.

Interpersonal effectiveness: For people who have endured extensive invalidation compounded by intense emotions, it can be difficult to advocate for themselves, to set limits, to repair relationships, and to consider the perspectives of others. This difficulty arises because their previous attempts have typically been unsuccessful. For example, say that some interaction is upsetting to you, and you tell the other person, and they then dismiss it. You haven't gotten your point across, or if you did, they dismissed it. You are further upset, because the situation was important to you. So, you raise your voice and express yourself more emphatically. The other person asks you why you are yelling at them. You feel that you can't win, and so you shut down. Then the other asks you why you aren't talking. These types of interactions tend to have the effect of reinforcing the idea that there is something wrong with you, which over time, is part of the path to self-loathing, and leads to difficulties in navigating relationships in an effective way.

Because interpersonal deficits typically arise from chronic invalidation, your most important task is that of self-validation. You recognize that your suffering makes sense given your emotional sensitivity and your early experiences, and that you can have compassion for yourself and that you can preserve your self-respect, even when others say that you are making a big deal about nothing or are rejecting your perspective.

The interpersonal effectiveness skills of DBT focus on you getting more of what you want. It allows you to set strong limits or boundaries that don't compromise your values, repair relationships, and teaches you how to accurately evaluate and consider other people's perspectives without destroying relationships, especially if their behavior is confusing to you, in order to reduce conflict.

Emotion regulation: How does a person learn to regulate their emotions? Unlike skills such as walking or riding a bike, which are commonly taught and celebrated in childhood, emotion regulation is rarely addressed directly in school, online courses, or even at home. Consider the developmental milestones parents celebrate: learning to walk, mastering the use of a spoon, or finally riding a bike without training wheels. These accomplishments are met with parental pride and encouragement. Yet, when it comes to managing emotions – such as fear or sadness – there is often a lack of similar guidance and recognition. Imagine a child who is afraid of the dark or upset over an ill grandparent. Rarely do we see the same level of encouragement for successfully managing these emotional challenges.

Additionally, parents might, intentionally or unintentionally, use their child's emotions to elicit the behaviors they want, further complicating the development of healthy emotional regulation. The absence of structured support in emotional regulation can leave you struggling with how to navigate your feelings effectively.

People who don't have difficulty regulating their sadness, anger, envy, and so on, are confused by those who don't know how to do so. If you haven't learned how to manage emotions, learning to do so can be lifesaving. The emotion regulation skill set teaches you the main aspects of emotion regulation:

a. It teaches about emotions, what they are and why we have them in the first place.

b. It teaches you how they manifest.

c. It teaches you how to validate how you are feeling.

d. It teaches you to discern between when emotions are justified and when they are not. What this means is whether the emotions fit the facts or not. For instance, fearing a rattlesnake on a hiking trail is a justified fear, because if it bites you, you could get seriously ill. Fearing a rattlesnake in a protected glass enclosure at the zoo is not justified as it cannot bite you, so the fear does not fit the facts. Now, if you fear the rattlesnake in each circumstance, your fear is what you feel, and so fear is valid. Only it is justified in the first situation and unjustified in the second.

e. It teaches you how to reduce your vulnerability to painful emotions and how to enhance wanted emotions. For instance, recognizing that not getting enough sleep and drinking excessive alcohol is a vulnerability factor for depression may seem obvious, but few of us ever truly recognize the link between these vulnerability factors and our emotional state.

f. It teaches that clarity and precision are important in learning to regulate your emotions. For instance, saying that you feel anger, sadness, or joy is clear. Saying that you are feeling "overwhelmed" tells others that you don't like how you are feeling; however, it is less precise and is an idea that represents a mixture of different emotions.

g. Finally, it teaches you what to do when you are experiencing an unwanted emotion. An example of such a skill is one known as the skill of opposite action. Here's how it works: Say you are feeling sad and want to isolate and stay in bed. The behavior of staying in bed does not generally make anyone feel happy, and certainly not in the long term. Doing opposite action is doing the opposite of your urge, in this case the urge to stay in bed and isolate, and so opposite would be to get up, take a shower, and call a friend.

THE SKILL OF OPPOSITE ACTION: I want to highlight the skill of opposite action as it is one of DBT's most powerful skills. Might it apply to tackling self-hatred? Conceptually it could work. For instance, say that because you feel self-hatred, you also feel that no decent person could ever like you. You go onto a dating app and accept anyone who expresses any interest in you and then date them even if they treat you poorly, feeling that it is the best that you can do, and that you deserve ill treatment. Opposite action would be rejecting people who are disrespectful and going on dates with people who have shared values and interests. Opposite action would include dressing up nicely for your date and accepting any kindness as genuine. It would also mean walking away from any request for behavior that crosses your values. I think that there is merit to the practice of opposite action for self-hatred; however, in my clinical experience, it does not help in the same way that it does for other emotions. This is because whereas the skill works in specific instances of emotional experience – such as a sudden burst of anger, sadness, disgust, envy and so on – because self-loathing is so deeply embedded, it rarely comes with a clearly discernable behavior, and so the way in which it might work is to be very clear about the specific behaviors that show up when self-hatred is active.

EXERCISE

Reflect on the behaviors that show up when you are experiencing particularly strong self-hatred.

ANSWER: Write down these behaviors and for each behavior, write down what opposite action would look like.

____

____

____

____

____

____

____

____

Hopefully by the time you have reached this part of the book, you are at least open to the idea that self-hatred is a construct that can shift a little and even begin to change. One practice that you could do that builds on the idea of opposite action is to do something nice for yourself each day. If you are willing to consider that you are not some terrible being and that you deserve a degree of kindness, start by being kind to yourself by doing something that makes you feel better. A bubble bath? A cup of hot chocolate? Going for a walk? Treating yourself to a new item of clothing?

EXERCISE

What are some things that you do not do for yourself because you feel undeserving?

YOUR ANSWER:

____

____

____

TASK: Pick from the list of self-kindness activities and do something nice for yourself at least once a week, and if you can, every day.

It's important to understand that DBT is not a magic elixir; it offers valuable tools but does not address every aspect of emotional distress on its own. Here are the reflections of one patient:

> *"I have engaged in a lot of outpatient DBT therapy. I view DBT skills as being a 'fake it till you make it' sort of paradigm. The skills help me regulate my emotions in the moment and make better decisions surrounding the use of maladaptive coping skills; however, they have yet to modify the core issues that inspire my BPD symptoms. I credit DBT with giving me the ability to be a functional adult human, but it has not made me happy or fulfilled, and certainly has not touched my self-hatred in a lasting manner. Because of this, I often feel like my life and my mental*

health progress is completely fake, and like I am tricking everyone into thinking that I'm stable and normal while secretly living a double life as a crazy/unstable person. I worry that I will never be able to be normal or happy in life and that I am doomed to constantly faking functionally while secretly being in a state of barely hanging on, one wrong move away from a future where I am destined to either kill myself or go insane."

Whereas the idea of "fake it till you make it" may work for many skills and contexts, the application of DBT to core self-loathing did not help this patient and this is consistent with my clinical experience. DBT has helped many of the people who have come to our program, but it has not dented self-hatred. It is possible that this is in part because it hasn't been tackled directly. The skills are critical for anyone who is suffering, but they are not enough. There is hope in integrating additional therapeutic approaches that address self-loathing more directly, but it's important to recognize that DBT alone is not a complete solution.

Mentalization-Based Therapy (MBT)

Mentalization-based therapy (MBT) is an evidence-based treatment that has been shown to be helpful for people who have BPD. It was developed by Drs. Peter Fonagy and Anthony Bateman who published the results of their first trial in 1999 (Bateman and Fonagy 1999). The approach is based on the idea that you are able to recognize and understand how your state of mind, and other people's state of mind, influences your and their behavior, and further, to distinguish between your own emotional state of mind and that of others.

For example, say that you work as a nurse-aid and live near the hospital. You are in your apartment and have just had dinner. You hear a knock at the door and your nurse friend has shown up unexpectedly. She barely says hello, says that she is ravenous and bizarrely, heads straight for your fridge and devours the leftover lasagna you were saving for tomorrow's lunch!

On the one hand you might find this behavior to be very rude and inconsiderate. A mentalizing approach would recognize that your nurse's state of mind makes her behavior understandable. We know that your friend is a nurse. One explanation could be that she is being rude, but you know her, it is unusual behavior for her. An alternative explanation could be that she had had an extremely long and busy shift, had not had a meal break, and was too exhausted to cook, and that because she was too tired and hungry to go home, that she came over to yours. Her behavior would make more sense given her state of mind. MBT focuses on helping people know and differentiate between their state of mind and someone else's.

There is very little written about MBT's approach to self-hatred; however, one case study described its application in a patient that they described thus (Drozek and Unruh 2022):

> Claire was a 30-year-old doctor whose emotions and behavior ...
>
> "oscillated unpredictably between intense anger toward others and self-hatred, once declaring, 'I am bad, disgusting, ugly, and worthless. No one wants to be with me, and that is never going to change.' Claire fantasized about suicide in these moments. She even wrote suicide letters to her family that remained unsent. By the time she reached residency, she had started cutting herself with razors."

The authors reflected on the progress that Claire had made and conclude: "Deeper understanding of her search for care led Claire to begin imagining how she might express emotional needs without becoming psychiatrically ill. When with friends, Claire spoke less about her psychiatric symptoms and more about work, relationships, and shared interests. Claire created a profile on a dating app and, to her great surprise, it was flooded with interest. Resuming dating after many years lifted her mood and provided a sense of satisfaction that came from moving toward her goal of having a stable long-term relationship. She threw away the razors she once saved for cutting 'just in case I needed them.' By the end of one year in MBT, Claire evinced notable functional improvements (e.g., improved attendance at work, no hospitalizations, no self-injury) as well as a subtle but notable shift in her experience of herself."

The researchers note that she had a "subtle but notable shift in her experience of herself, and although we don't know if she experienced less self-hatred, it does appear that she was able to engage in her life, in her work, with her friends and romantic partners in a more meaningful way, and we might conclude that her self-loathing reduced."

Schema Therapy

Schema therapy is a type of therapy that targets *schemas* which is a term used to describe unhealthy patterns of thinking that can cause you to engage in unhealthy or maladaptive behavior. They can be a pattern that causes you to struggle to maintain healthy adult relationships. These patterns, or schemas, develop during childhood, and particularly in children whose emotional and physical needs weren't met. In schema theory, unhealthy patterns can also develop in children who were overindulged or whose parents did not set developmentally appropriate limits. The theory is that once a person reaches adulthood, these schemas then influence a person's thoughts and actions in negative ways, leading to behaviors such as avoidance, overcompensation, or excessive self-sacrifice, behaviors which, in turn, negatively impact relationships and emotional well-being.

Schema therapy identifies 18 different schemas. One of the schemas pertinent to this book is termed "Defectiveness and Shame."

This schema is driven by the core beliefs such as, "There is something fundamentally wrong with me," "I am not loveable," "I am inherently flawed." Schema posits that it develops in a childhood when there is childhood abuse, neglect, or rejection. Then, the way that the child was treated caused the child to conclude that they were at fault or because there was something bad, shameful, or flawed about the child. Then, because children don't have the capacity to see that parents or caregivers are at fault, they interpret their abusive or neglectful treatment as being a reflection of the flaws and their own behavior.

As you've read in previous accounts, the child might say something like: "If I was a better child and if there wasn't something wrong with me, I would be loved." From a schema perspective, the shame that is internalized is termed toxic shame. Schema theory recognizes that a person can develop this schema even if there wasn't any obvious maltreatment. Even if a person had every material comfort, they can still develop this pattern if they didn't have a person who paid attention and validated their thoughts and feelings in childhood.

The defectiveness and shame schema is characterized by a profound effect on relationships in that it can prevent establishing intimate connections. Because you feel that you are so flawed, you don't want to get close to anyone. One of my patients told me that self-hatred is like some genetic illness. *"You know there are some genetic illnesses that you don't want to pass on to children, so you don't get close to anyone. I worry that I will pass on my flaws onto the other person and even to my children if it ever got that far. But it will never get that far because if I let anyone see who I really am, they won't want to be with me."*

Other than relationships, this schema has a significant impact on emotional health and sense of self and is one of the primary schemas that drives depression. The self-loathing and self-criticism are considered to cause depression.

The behaviors seen as typical in this schema include:

- hyper-sensitivity to criticism and rejection
- self-loathing
- tolerating mistreatment by others
- taking responsibility and blame for problems you didn't cause
- picking critical partners
- staying in dysfunctional relationships for fear that you'll never find someone else

Given that schema therapy focuses so much on the kinds of ideas and constructs that are tied to self-loathing, it might be a useful approach to address self-loathing, However, like all the other therapies and theories mentioned, schema therapy has no published studies on its impact on chronic self-hatred.

Bottom-line: There are commonalties to all of the aforementioned therapies, and ones that can be of use to tackling self-hatred. They all recognize that self-loathing has its roots in early childhood. That it is learned through repeated interactions that leave the child concluding that they are flawed individuals, and that identifying and challenging the negative core beliefs and exposing them as false conclusions are key to overcoming them. Nevertheless, the approaches have not been tested in core self-hatred.

In the next chapter, we'll review what makes tackling self-hatred so difficult. I include it to validate the challenge that lies ahead, and why many of the well-meaning recommendations of friends, family, and therapists are not as helpful as they intend. I also include it, because even though there are some initial barriers to a path toward self-acceptance and compassion, they are all ones that you can overcome.

Chapter 12

Why Is Self-Hatred So Hard to Tackle?

In my nearly 25 years since I arrived at McLean Hospital, I have seen people heal from some significant mental health challenges. I have seen patients who have recovered from severe anorexia, depression, bipolar disorder, substance misuse, and so on. I have seen people stop making suicide attempts, stop cutting, stop using the drugs and alcohol that debilitated their lives. I have seen advances in the understanding of treatment of different conditions and the introduction of new approaches, therapies such as DBT, medications such as ketamine, and neuromodulating technologies such as trans cranial stimulation of the brain. And yet, it all my years, self-hatred has not been addressed in any systemized way.

For people reading this, I want to recognize that the mental health community of providers has not addressed this debilitating experience. I am hopeful that by bringing self-hatred into increased public awareness, that more research will be undertaken, and more therapists will address it. However, this book is not primarily written for researchers or therapists. It is written for the person with lived experience. I want to recognize that you might have been struggling with self-hatred for a long time and that reducing it has likely been difficult or felt like an impossible task.

In this context, I want to start by addressing why it may have been difficult to tackle self-hatred. Many of these barriers might be ones that resonate with your experience, and others could be ones that you had not considered. By bringing them up I am naming them as possible obstacles and then proposing some ideas that might help overcome them.

Therapists Don't Ask

If you've been in therapy, you've likely experienced an initial psychiatric evaluation. Think about the interviews that you have had. If you haven't been in therapy but are considering it, here's what to expect. These questions will be familiar to those who've had therapy and informative for those who haven't.

The standard intake interview is this list of common questions. If you want, you could fill this out. As you review these, think about what set of questions are missing from this intake form.

The first set of questions is about who you are, and what your social circumstances are:

- Your name
- Age
- For adults: relationship status and children (if any)
- Your occupation or your level of education
- Your living situation (where, with whom)
- Who is in your family (parents, siblings)
- Other health care providers (past and present, including other therapists, psychiatrists, primary care physician)

The next set of questions is about what brought you to therapy:

- We start with direct questions, such as: "What brings you to therapy?"
- Therapists might ask who recommended them? (Another therapist, a medical doctor, a family member, an insurance company list)
- We then allow the person to share their story and try to do so without interrupting them! Some of us have the bad habit of interrupting as soon as patients start talking.
- Next, we focus on their symptoms, typically over the past month, but these may have lasted longer.

- We then ask about any past psychiatric history, and if there have been medication trials.

The next set of questions is digging further into specific symptoms, such as:

- **Sleep.** We want to know about the quality of sleep. (important in mood disorders)
  - When do you go to bed?
  - When do you fall asleep?
  - Amount of sleep.
  - What time do you get up?
  - Do you wake up during the night?
  - We might ask about snoring if we are assessing for sleep apnea, which is related to depression.
  - Do you ever experience nightmares? (often related to trauma)
- **Interests:** We want to know about the things that bring you joy and pleasure, or loss of pleasure.
  - Hobbies
  - Regular activities
  - Interests
- **Guilt:** Standard interview, particularly if screening for depression is to ask about feeling guilty.
- **Energy:** We want to know if your energy level has gone up or down.
- **Attention and concentration:** These can be impacted by depression, anxiety, ADHD, and other mental health conditions.
- **Appetite, eating behaviors, and changes in weight:** These are particularly relevant for eating disorders and mood disorders, and may be a consequence of the side-effects of psychiatric medications.
- **Suicidal thoughts and behaviors.**

- **Self-harm behaviors.**
- **Irritability: Common in bipolar disorder.**
- **Assess for grandiose or paranoid delusions:** More common in bipolar disorder or psychotic disorders.
- **Asses for hallucinations:** These are essential questions for psychotic disorders such as schizophrenia, or as a consequence of certain drugs, or perhaps because of a neurological disorder such as certain types of epilepsy.
- **Assess for obsessions and compulsions:** These questions are relevant if obsessive compulsive disorder (OCD) is suspected.
- **Trauma symptoms:** Such as flashbacks, intrusive memories, trauma nightmares, a strong startle reflex.
- **Substance use:** Including alcohol, tobacco, cannabis, stimulants, and also the misuse of prescriptions drugs.
- **Relevant medical history:** Many medical conditions can cause, aggravate, or worsen mental health. For instance, chronic illness, traumatic brain injury, the side-effects of medications used to treat medical conditions.
- **Past trauma history:** Including physical, emotional, verbal, and sexual abuse.
- **Developmental history:** Including schooling, early development, history of learning difficulties, employment history, and difficulties at work.
- **Relationship history:** Including relationships with family, friends, coworkers, as well as an assessment of your support system.
- **Faith and religion:** If pertinent.
- **Family history of mental illness:** This is particularly relevant if there is a strong family history of mood, psychotic, and substance use disorders.

What is the point of my highlighting these assessment questions? If you have ever had a mental health evaluation, you are very familiar with all these questions. **What is missing in the multiple questions, is any assessment of self-hatred. It's remarkable a symptom or experience that is so closely linked to suicidal behavior is not asked about.**

Of course, there are exceptions, and some therapists do ask about how a person sees themselves, but in my experience and in my training, any direct questions about self-hatred are very rare. How does a therapist address a symptom if we don't ask about it?

I know that until recently, I was guilty of not asking about self-hatred, even though it is something that patients have suffered with for such a long time. I wanted to make sure that it hadn't been assessed in the patients who helped me with the ideas in this book. I asked them if they had ever been asked about self-loathing. You don't have to be a researcher to notice the common theme:

Answer 1: No

Answer 2: Never

Answer 3: No

Answer 4: No one has ever asked me about self-loathing

Answer 5: No

Answer 6. No. I had to tell my therapist about it.

Answer 7: No

Answer 8: No

Answer 9: No, but I also never brought it up

Answer 10: No. Anyway I thought my therapist hated me and I just didn't want it confirmed.

WHAT YOU CAN DO TO OVERCOME THIS OBSTACLE: If you experience self-hatred and your therapist doesn't ask about it, tell them you struggle with it in the same way that you would tell them about any other symptom.

Avoidance

> "The more you try to avoid suffering, the more you suffer, because smaller and more insignificant things begin to torture you, in proportion to your fear of being hurt. The one who does most to avoid suffering is, in the end, the one who suffers most."
>
> —Thomas Merton, *The Seven Storey Mountain*

Marsha Linehan, the developer of DBT and guided by contemplative practices, said something very similar: "Avoidance of suffering leads to worse suffering."

In my clinical experience many patients avoid wanting to talk about, or be willing to consider and tackle, the experience of self-hatred. There are two main reasons for this avoidance. The first is that because it can feel so unchangeable, it can feel like a waste of time in therapy. The second is the belief that talking about self-hatred will be so painful, that the suffering isn't worth it. Let's look at some key concepts.

Avoidance and Escape

Avoidance refers to behaviors that show up when you either won't, or refuse to, enter into an experience or situation. Escape refers to the behavior of leaving, or removing yourself, from an unwanted experience as soon as you can.

Avoidance and escape are natural mechanisms for coping with many potentially dangerous situations and under those circumstances, they are adaptive survival behaviors. For instance, if you are severely allergic to peanuts, it makes sense that you would want to avoid peanuts. Or, if you fell off a boat in the Florida Everglades and you saw an alligator, it would make sense that you would want to escape as soon as possible. Clearly there are many situations where active avoidance is clearly to your advantage, because not doing so could result in significant harm.

Different to the peanut and the boating example, when it comes to treatment and therapy, avoidance and escape as a response to stressful therapy topics can keep you trapped in a cycle of suffering because the issue is never addressed and dealt with. This is particularly true when you are avoiding addressing a situation where there is no longer an actual threat of harm to you. Unfortunately, the problem is that once the avoidance and escape behavior has been learned, repeated, and reinforced over many years, it can become a habit which is no longer tied to the reason the avoidance started in the first place. And you should know, you might not be the only one avoiding the topic. Many therapists avoid talking to their patients about difficult issues, because either (i) they don't want to bring up stressful topics or (ii) they don't want to experience their patient's suffering.

Before considering how avoidance applies to tackling self-hated, let's look at some common avoidance strategies. Consider each of these and think whether they apply to you:

1. **Situational avoidance:** This is the most common type of avoidance, and refers to staying away from people, places, things, or activities that cause you distress. For instance, say you have a relative who used to blame and belittle you and whose words made you feel worse about yourself. Avoiding going to his house would be an example of situational avoidance.

   Exercise: Does this apply to me? If so, an example of this is:

   ____

   ____

2. **Somatic avoidance:** Somatic means *body*, and in this context, it means avoiding body sensations. This type of avoidance is often connected to situational avoidance; however, it more specifically refers to avoiding situations that elicit a physical response that can

feel like anxiety or stress. The common somatic sensations include: a racing heart, tingling sensations in your fingers, nausea or feeling a pit in your stomach. Different from situational avoidance where you avoid specific situations, with somatic situations you avoid activities that cause physical responses. For example, going on a roller coaster may not be a situation that caused you stress in the past, but because it causes your heart to race and you feel a pit in your stomach, you avoid the roller coaster in order to avoid the physical or somatic sensations.

Exercise: Does this apply to me? If so, an example of this is:

____

____

3. **Cognitive avoidance:** This is avoidance that happens inside your mind. For example, say you have a thought or memory of a hurtful relative. Distracting from the memory or telling yourself not to think about the person, or to focus on something else, would be an example of cognitive avoidance.

   Exercise: Does this apply to me? If so, an example of this is:

   ____

   ____

4. **Protective avoidance:** This type of avoidance is more common in people with OCD and includes doing actions in your physical space to help you feel safe; for instance, compulsively cleaning your kitchen as a way to avoid the distressing thought that you might get infected with some illness caused by a dirty kitchen would be protective avoidance.

   Exercise: Does this apply to me? If so, an example of this is:

   ____

   ____

5. **Substitution avoidance:** This type of avoidance is using a substitute behavior instead of doing the behavior that causes you suffering. For instance, rather than experiencing sadness and fear by calling a sick relative, you substitute calling your relative by using drugs, or alcohol, in order to avoid the sadness or fear.

   Exercise: Does this apply to me? If so, an example of this is:

   ____

   ____

Self-Loathing and Avoidance

It is totally natural to avoid thinking about, being around, and remembering the things that remind you of painful experiences, and this is even more so if these experiences were traumatic. However, avoidance of suffering leads to more suffering because the experience isn't addressed. Emotional avoidance takes a psychic toll as it is exhausting to actively keep avoiding.

ANALOGY: Imagine that you had a toothache. You decide to not go to the dentist but it is sore, so you mask the pain through taking heavy-duty painkillers. Sure, the pain goes away temporarily, but you haven't dealt with what is causing the pain in the first place. Eventually the pain will come back, and if it's an infected tooth, the painkillers can't cure it so the infection will spread, and the problem becomes far bigger than just that one tooth.

In this case, targeting the avoidance should be a key focus in treatment.

WHAT YOU CAN DO TO OVERCOME THIS OBSTACLE: Expanding on what you have just read, are you using avoidance or escape behaviors as a way to not address the self-hatred? If so, how?

____

____

____

____

Certainty That It Can't Change

It goes without saying that most people who seek mental health treatment do so because they are struggling in some way and they believe that therapy, with or without medication, will help reduce whatever mental state is causing their distress. Believing that therapy and medication can help makes sense, because research shows that treatments such as cognitive behavioral therapy (CBT) can help for depression and that exposure and response prevention (ERP) can reduce OCD symptoms, and that mood stabilizers can help with bipolar disorder and so on.

When it comes to self-hatred however, and as others have expressed elsewhere in this book, few who experience it believe that it can change. Here are some reflections on this belief:

Answer 1. A person who has just started to tackle self-hatred: *"I tried to use concrete evidence to challenge the self-loathing thoughts but that never worked for very long. For example – even if I had tons of evidence that my boss didn't hate me (she gave me positive feedback often, brought me coffee all the time, genuinely cared about how I was feeling, wanted to promote me to general manager) I was still very convinced that those were just 'flukes' or that she was just being nice because she had to be. So, I have read and answered your questions as well as I could have but it was hard to answer questions about how it has shifted because I don't feel like it has or ever will. (But maybe that is just my mindset right now, I'm sure other people have different experiences.)"*

Answer 2: *"Telling me to do self-compassion – just telling me to do that – yes it is superficial but also simply unrealistic. With self-hatred often (or at least for me) also comes the feeling of not deserving anything good ... so how are you telling me to go do some self-care? Why would I do that? (I understand the premise, just pointing out the challenge when filled with such deep self-hatred.) To 'get better' I have to create a life worth living by decreasing suffering, but I don't believe I deserve anything good and feel the constant need to punish myself. I just don't believe it so what's even the point in trying?"*

WHAT YOU CAN DO TO OVERCOME THIS OBSTACLE: Are you certain that your self-hatred can't change? If so, write about it. There is significant research that shows that simply naming your emotional experience reduces the impact of the emotion. For instance, saying "I am angry," will reduce the level of anger. Naming your worst concerns is a way to start to conquer them.

____

____

____

____

____

____

____

Comparisons: The Ever-Present Trigger

One of my patients told me that what got in the way of working on her self-hatred was her experience of being compared to her ever-present, one-year-older sister. She said that coming home after school and hearing about her sister's grades and accomplishments were a constant reminder of what a flaw she is. This is what she told me: *"Comparisons impact my self-hatred a lot, and it increases the level of self-hatred because the comparisons lead to feelings of being less than, therefore not as good as a person. The level of intensity of the self-hatred depends on the subject, but all comparisons lead to self-hatred. For example, comparisons with my sister, even though she is my favorite person in the world, lead to higher levels of self-hatred whereas comparisons with people like my teachers don't produce the same level of self-hatred. But it also happens when I compare myself to myself. Let's say I am writing a term paper. If I exceed standards one of two things could happen.*

The first is that I might feel okay or 2, and this happens more frequently, I might be set up for failure because maybe the standards will be raised, and therefore I will have to be even better of a person, which I'm not capable of."

Certainly, there will be many others who are better at many things than we are. Why does this need to perpetuate the self-loathing?

> "Today you are You, that is truer than true. There is no one alive who is Youer than You."
>
> —Dr. Seuss

No one can be better at being you than you can at being you. Now, if you say that you don't want to be you, what are the elements of youness that you can work on? Remember that your future needs you. Your past does not, and in this moment, you can start to see that no one can make you a "better person." Only you can. Comparing yourself to others rarely helps. Every single person on Earth has things that they are better at, and that they are worse at, than others. And even those who are the best at things, will one day stop being the best. And you can be grateful that you don't have to be the best 100-meter runner, painter, writer, card player, pianist, mathematician, and so on. All you have to work toward is the best version of who you are. And in truth, in any given moment, given your circumstances and vulnerability factors, you actually are the best version of you! At the same time it is also true that you need to work harder and try new ways to overcome the barriers to self-compassion, whether you erected those barriers or someone else did.

WHAT YOU CAN DO TO OVERCOME THIS OBSTACLE: Are comparisons feeding into your self-hatred? If so, what are the comparisons you are making? Can you compare yourself to the child who was hurt? Can you see how you would address the hurt today?

____

____

____

____

Praise Does Not Work

Over the years, I have asked patients who experience self-hatred if being praised by the people they love is ever helpful. When it comes to reducing self-hatred, the resounding answer is NO. Here is what one patient told me: *"Experiences where I receive positive affirmation tend to lessen the intensity of self-loathing temporarily, but it doesn't fundamentally change it or get rid of it. These experiences have to be genuine(i.e., not said out of obligation) and not too intense (i.e., overly positive in an inauthentic way) for me to be able to internalize them. However, it is very difficult for me to accept praise because my self-loathing makes me feel like I don't deserve it and that I'm a horrible person if I don't hate myself constantly."*

Another one told me: *"Yup. I always feel like they're lying to me, especially my parents, and that they are just saying it to make me feel better. But even my friends. The other day, I went to my friend's house and there was a girl I liked, and the first things she said to me was 'Hi you! You look great!' I wanted to tell her: 'Really? Because I feel like shit, and you don't have to be nice to me.' My friend tells me that the girl likes me, but I don't believe it. And it is worse when they praise me. I just don't believe it."*

WHAT YOU CAN DO TO OVERCOME THIS OBSTACLE: Write down the problem that you have with praise. Next, if it is clear that people are praising you simply to make you feel better about yourself, you can acknowledge their intention but let them know that it is not helpful. Further, if they do something that is helpful, let them know that as well. Finally, accept praise as a true reflection of others' perspective because sometimes you are simply fabulous!

The bottom line is that when you are not asked about it, when you avoid talking about it, when you don't believe that it can change, and when the praise of others feels untrue, tackling self-hatred is difficult. When therapists don't ask about it, it creates a gap in understanding and treatment, leaving you feeling isolated in your struggle. Avoiding the topic yourself can perpetuate feelings of inadequacy, making it harder to confront and work through these emotions. If you don't believe that change is possible, it can feel like a hopeless endeavor, and this mindset can become a self-fulfilling prophecy. The belief that you are stuck with these feelings forever can prevent you from seeking help or trying new approaches that could lead to improvement. To tackle self-hatred, you must bring it into the open, both in therapeutic settings and in your self-reflection. Acknowledging its presence is the first step toward addressing it. Believing in the possibility of change, even if it feels difficult, can open the door to new strategies and perspectives. This belief is not naïvete. There have been things that you believed in the past that you no longer do. Beliefs can change. Learning to accept and believe in the praise and positive feedback from others can help shift your self-perception over time. Ultimately, tackling self-hatred requires a multifaceted approach. It's about creating an environment, both within yourself and with the support of others, where self-compassion and growth are possible.

Chapter 13

Reflections of Therapists

I have included this chapter because I want to highlight the point that we as therapists are not trained to ask about self-hatred, and when it comes up, we aren't taught how to treat or address it. And this is an important point because even though self-hatred is far more common in the patients that I and my colleagues see in our clinical practice, we ourselves seldom ask about it and certainly have few ideas as to how to address it. I reached out to some of my colleagues and asked them the questions that follow. If you are in therapy and your therapist doesn't ask you about it, you are not alone. Most people with self-hatred aren't asked about it, and as we just reviewed in the previous chapter, if you are in therapy, it is completely reasonable to talk to your therapist about it and its impact on your life.

Questions for therapists:

1. Do you see patients who have told you they hate themselves? If so, what percentage of your patients would you say hate themselves? By this I mean a core enduring self-loathing, not just something that is transient.
2. Did you ever ask about self-loathing as a part of your comprehensive initial evaluation?
3. Can you give me some examples about how it manifests in the patients who recognize that they struggle with self-loathing?
4. How has it impacted your patients' lives?

5. Have you ever directly addressed it in therapy? If yes, how, if not, why not? If you tried, what were the challenges?

Here is how they responded.

THERAPIST 1: (DBT Residential Unit)

1. Absolutely. I would say that at least 80% of my patients who meet criteria for BPD experience core, enduring self-loathing. To them, it feels extremely static and unchangeable. Among patients who do not have BPD the percentage is likely lower, although still common to the extent that when I have a patient who does not experience self-loathing, it is noticeable and somewhat relieving as a therapist. I would estimate that among those who do not have BPD, the enduring self-loathing would be closer to 20%, although transient self-loathing would likely be around 80%.
2. I typically do not formally assess self-loathing because it usually becomes abundantly clear as soon as you start talking to the patient. To be honest, I tend to avoid the topic early on, as it can send us down a rabbit hole, and it can sometimes be destabilizing.
3. I find that those who have difficulty experiencing hope for the future often also experience a deep sense of self-loathing. One case being a young woman who felt that having any hope for the future would be tempting fate. For example, she might say something like, "But if I think, 'Okay, maybe it won't turn out so bad' then the universe will do something terrible to put me back in my place." The very idea of experiencing anything positive or hopeful evokes a deep sense of fear. She often explained that hating herself was the price she paid to live in this world.

   If others caught on that she felt anything other than self-hatred, she would be a pariah.

   Perhaps not so ironically, another presentation tends to be displays of narcissism. I vividly remember a teenaged young woman I'll call Amy. I was reviewing a "family chain" of her suicide attempt.

(*Author's note:* A family chain is an analysis of each family member sharing a step-by-step assessment of what happened in a situation; in this case a suicide attempt.) Immediately before the actual suicide attempt Amy was screaming at her sister and mother, telling them what terrible people they were, and how she couldn't wait to get away from their toxicity. She emphasized the wonderful life she would have without them "dragging me down." Weeks later, during family therapy, Amy tearfully told her mother how much she hated herself, and how in that moment the self-hatred became too much to bear. Amy's mother expressed genuine shock. Explaining that her assessment had been that Amy hated them while simultaneously feeling wonderfully about her own self. Amy emphatically discounted this, emphasizing the intense loneliness she experiences, and then envy that burns within her when she watches her mother and sister seemingly breeze through their own lives.

Finally, patients who have experienced early childhood trauma, particularly sexual abuse, appear to experience a particularly strong and persistent self-loathing. I frequently hear these patients describe themselves as "defective." Their explanations for their trauma tend to be extremely judgmental such as: "I'm just a slut" (despite being seven years old at the time of the abuse), or "I deserved it, I was a really bad kid," or "I was already worthless, that's why it happened. Who cares?" Clinically, the only thing I have seen turn this self-loathing around has been DBT-PE. (*Author's note:* DBT-PE is a treatment for people with emotion dysregulation and PTSD. It combines the use of DBT [see Chapter 11] and a technique known as prolonged exposure, which has been shown to be effective in treating PTSD.)

4. It has impacted nearly every moment of their lives. It's difficult to put into words and seems impossible to quantify how profoundly hating yourself can affect your life. It affects their hope for the future, how likely they are to try something new, their ability to engage in fulfilling relationships with others, and very often leads to extremely self-destructive behaviors.

5. I remember learning in my training to "forget self-esteem and focus on self-efficacy." I have found this to be the most effective approach. Discussing self-loathing at length can send us down an unproductive, and often very frustrating rabbit hole. I tend to address self-loathing with exposure tasks that often do not seem targeted at self-loathing at all. Some examples may be requiring a patient who has not functioned typically in many years, to get a job, assigning a patient to buy clothes that fit them properly, or encouraging a patient who won't express her needs in a relationship, for example, to ask to go to a particular restaurant despite it not being a preferred place for their partner. As these tasks start to add up, I ask questions such as, "How did you feel after your first shift at work? What was it like to not feel uncomfortable in your jeans today? Did you think you'd be able to do it?" I have also very consciously shifted away from saying, "I feel proud of you," and have started saying, "I hope you feel proud of yourself." I have noticed this to be a very effective method of reinforcing patients' achievements and encouraging continued exposures. As the exposures and functioning increase, it seems that self-loathing begins to decrease.

Reflection: I find a few things interesting about my colleague's response. The first is that there is consistency between her noting that her patient's self-loathing started very early, age seven in her patient's case, and the answers that my patients provided as to early onset. The second is that she fears bringing up the topic, and in fact avoids it, because she is worried that it could destabilize her patients.

My colleague is courageous in admitting this, and she is not alone in avoiding the topic. This approach, avoidance, is also one that historically plagued many other disorders. In the past, clinicians would not talk about a cancer diagnosis or AIDS. They would use terms like "the C word," or "the virus." Without addressing symptoms and diagnoses directly, they will stay in the shadows, and we won't know what to do. Many therapists share my colleague's fear that they will be heading down the rabbit hole of spiraling futility, however as with many other symptoms, such as talking about suicidal thoughts, without addressing self-loathing, the experience will stay buried in the rabbit hole.

ACTION ITEM: Your therapist might not ask you about self-hatred, or know how to help you, or be worried themselves about bringing it up. Bring it up. If it is impacting your life, it is relevant to therapy.

Remember, discussing difficult emotions, including self-hatred, is a crucial part of therapy. Therapists are trained to handle difficult conversations. If it helps, you can write down the key points in a diary and bring the diary to therapy to open up the conversation. Also, ideally you should bring it up at the beginning of a session when there is ample time to discuss it fully. Don't be afraid to ask the therapist for their thoughts and feedback on how you can work together to address self-hatred. One thing that I have noticed with my patients is that while the initial conversations were hard, the more we talked about it, the easier they became and the more progress we made.

THERAPIST 2: (Eating Disorder Residential)

1. I work on an eating disorder unit, and I would say around 15–20% of patients that I see on the unit have said that they fundamentally hate themselves.
2. I have never asked about self-loathing in an intake, nor to my knowledge have any of my colleagues. We sometimes ask about self-esteem, but not always.
3. I have noticed that it typically manifests in anger – when a patient feels threatened that another person is criticizing their character in any way or offering constructive feedback (on our unit, this could look like a staff member redirecting a comment or behavior), it leads to emotional dysregulation/lashing out on the individual. The patient is incredibly sensitive to criticism as it reinforces the feeling that they are fundamentally a bad person. I have noticed that they tend to seek out irrational signs to confirm the validity of their self-hatred.

4. I have found self-loathing deeply interferes with the ability to recover from mental health diagnoses, such as an eating disorder or OCD, as the feeling that they are fundamentally unworthy is so consuming that it shatters any motivation to make behavioral changes, or to accept that they are worthy of a life worth living. I have also noticed that it impacts relationships and career choices, where patients tend to become involved in an abusive relationship or stuck in an unsatisfying job.
5. Yes, I have tried to address it. CBT techniques like cognitive restructuring or cognitive reframing have historically been unhelpful. A patient once described it as "lying to my brain." Even reframing smaller, more specific self-critical thoughts tend to have a low believability rating. I have also not found cognitive diffusion to be helpful, as it is difficult for patients to diffuse the feeling of self-hatred. I try to have patients use more specific language when describing how they feel rather than "I hate myself" or "I want to die" which has been somewhat effective, yet they struggle to isolate specific thoughts that contribute to self-loathing. Mindfulness and the practice of self-compassion/instilling the hope of change has been most effective.

Reflection: Therapist 2 works in a very different context than therapist 1 does. If we take their answers to question 1, the percentage of people struggling with core self-loathing on a unit treating people with eating disorders is lower than on one treating people with BPD; HOWEVER, do we actually know that? Is there research that supports that the level of self-hatred is different? Clearly we need more research.

And once again, without explicitly asking about self-loathing, their answers to the statistics are at best, guesses, although informed guesses. Both therapists, just like many therapists I ask, and just as was my own practice, have not historically asked about self-loathing. Then, and not surprisingly, both therapists note that for their group of patients the sense of hope for a purposeful future is eroded if not shattered by the experience of self-hatred.

THERAPIST 3: (DBT Partial Hospital Program)

1. I work in a hospital and have a small private practice. Two of my thirteen private patients have deep seated hatred about themselves, that feels intractable. So about 15%? I have three other patients that talk/talked about hating themselves a lot – but not their whole essence/being. They hate a lot of what they do, or who they are, or how they come across – but these three feel different than the two others. I think all 13 patients have talked about hating themselves or some part of themselves at various points in therapy.

2. I don't actually – but maybe I should start asking about self-loathing. It always seems to come up organically. Usually when I am doing chain analysis of behavior. (*Author's note:* A chain analysis is a DBT tool where a therapist reviews a step-by-step account as to why a patient did a certain behavior. This is thoughts and emotions. Often, a behavior might happen because of self-loathing, or self-loathing can occur as a consequence of the behavior.)

3. My first patient is a college kid, who has been in different therapies for a long time. Their primary diagnosis is depression and anxiety. Although they are not self-destructive, they have long-standing self-hatred. Truly, truly hates everything about themselves. It's almost impossible to get them to say one kind, even neutral thing about themselves. There is such deep shame with them that they struggle to open up about anything deep/personal in therapy. I think because they hate themselves so much, they cannot understand how I also won't hate them (or be disgusted by, or angry at, or judge them) – so they keep therapy at very superficial levels. And when they do start to open up, they become so intensely emotional, they quickly package it all up and shut down. This then leads to them hating themselves even more *because* they've shut down and can't open up to me.

   My second patient is a high school grad hoping to start college in the fall. She also has a long history of treatment – including hospitalizations. She also has a history of depression and anxiety and many traits of BPD. She has struggled with self-injury and suicidal behavior. We just started working more intensely on her self-hatred in therapy, and she has identified three themes: her looks, her intelligence, and that she is annoying. She is not a super psychologically minded or insightful kid, so she struggles to give me context around how this all shows up. She keeps things super vague in therapy, which makes therapy not move that much. She's also not super bought into therapy, so I do wonder how motivated she is to target this. But we have to tackle this.

4. For the first patient, the impact on her is that she is miserable. Despite this, she is functioning – doing well in college (above and beyond actually), good grades, holds to all their appointments, has friends, but is so consumed with self-hatred. And so, even when she is thriving, and right now she is thriving more than ever in her life, she can't see the positive. She can't give herself credit for thriving.

The second patient is struggling, but I'm not sure if it's about self-hatred, mostly because it's hard to get a solid conceptualization of her. She's a "failure to launch" kid who often states that her depression gets her out of doing things, even when I believe she is more capable. (*Author's note:* Although "failure to launch" is not a formal diagnosis, it is used by the mental health profession to describe an older teen/young adult who is struggling with the transition to adulthood. It describes the inability or difficulty that the young person has when they try to leave home and support themselves.) She is definitely anxious and depressed, and I think she actually does know what to do but something gets in the way of doing things and so her parents step up to the plate each time and do for her. This is where I feel that she's not super bought in to change all this. I think the self-hatred mostly shows up around school, which leads to such anxiety/comparison thoughts about others, then to avoidance, and then to complete depression where she can't leave her bed.

5. In terms of addressing self-hatred, for my first patient, we've tried many things, like, checking the facts, acceptance, extending – nothing seems to work. As of now, our approach has been "just keep doing effective behaviors, and not pay attention to the hatred thoughts," because they are functioning well despite the self-loathing. She is pretty willful about letting go of these beliefs about herself, so doesn't seem to do some of the above skills wholeheartedly. This might just be because she is convinced that it cannot change. We've tried going about this in other ways – more exposures around emotions, with my hope that this could eventually get her to talk about the hatred thoughts and her rationale for them in more detail. As to how they developed, I don't have enough info on how they all developed.

For my second kid, we have just started to target it – started by gathering data (she's journaling about self-loathing experiences). We have started to use more check the facts and other skills. There are a lot of crises in her life, and we are constantly putting out fires, so I can imagine that we end up getting derailed because something more pressing comes up. (*Author's note:* Check the facts is a DBT skill. The focus is on the factual observable events of the situation. The reason to check the facts is that under many circumstances, the facts aren't what cause distress. Rather, more commonly it is the interpretation of the facts, the situation, the thoughts, or the emotions that cause distress. By sticking to the facts rather than the interpretation, our minds become clearer, and we are more capable of dealing with the situation.)

As you can see, even though many therapists recognize that they have patients who struggle with self-hatred, it is not a common part of their initial assessment. The topic tends to come up in the course of therapy, and when it does, the therapists don't exactly know what to do about it. Recognizing this gap is an important first step, and it opens up opportunities for more focused conversations and effective interventions as you continue your therapeutic journey.

So, you are not alone in feeling uncertain about what to do. You might wonder, "If the experts don't have all the answers, what can I do?" It's a valid question, but you have more power than you realize to change your self-hatred. Also, until you ask your therapist, you don't actually know that they don't know what to do. Many are trained in the types of therapies we reviewed in Chapter 11 and will have some ideas that could work with certain negative core beliefs. In the next chapter, we will explore the ideas and strategies of people who have overcome, or are in the process of overcoming, self-hatred.

Chapter 14

Advice from Those with Lived Experience

"You yourself, as much as anybody in the entire universe, deserve your love and affection."

—Buddha

We've just reviewed what research shows about the impact of the major therapies on reducing the experience of self-hatred, and also reviewed some of the major obstacles. Given that, at present, there is very little evidence that these therapies have much impact on self-hatred, I cover ideas in this chapter that my patients and I have explored and highlight the ones that they felt were helpful. Many of my patients have said that they were happy to share these ideas with others because they don't want others to suffer as much as they have. You are not alone in this journey, even if it has felt that way for a long time.

Here are their lived experience tested ideas.

Being Asked About It!

Many of the patients who shared their experience of self-hatred with me expressed surprise and even shock that I was asking about self-loathing. "No one has ever asked me about it before. I didn't even know that it was a thing to ask about it." When I sent my patients the list of questions in Chapter 3, I specifically asked them what they thought about being asked the questions, in terms of whether they helped or not. Here are some of their answers.

Answer 1: *"I think most of the questions were helpful to prompt purposeful thinking about this, especially questions about when/how self-hatred started and how it has impacted my life. I don't usually think of self-loathing from that kind of zoomed-out perspective, and it was insightful to think about it as a pattern that I have dealt with most of my life. I blame myself frequently but when I realize that I had the same tendencies when I was 6 or 7, I wish I had more self-compassion for my younger/current self."*

Answer 2: *"I have been in and out of treatment for 16 years. No one has ever asked me that question. Are you kidding me? What? It blows my mind."*

ACTION TASK: If your therapist has not asked you about self-hatred, commit to bringing it up at your next session. My next appointment is _______(date and time). I commit to bring it up at that appointment.

Focusing on the Concept of Future You

> "Thinking deeply about your choices and actions from the stance of your future self can serve as both a motivational and a corrective force."
>
> —Cheryl Strayed

What is the concept of future you and how can it help tackle self-loathing? At its most basic level, it is the concept of you a minute from now, tomorrow, next week, next month, next year, and so on.

EXERCISES: Imagine a future you, a you that has succeeded in accomplishing at least one of your goals.

1. What are the tasks you need to do *now*, so that future you is successful? Are you preparing the present you to be that future person?

____

____

____

2. How are you caring about present you in ways that future you will look back and appreciate your present efforts?

____

____

3. Is mistreating and hating the you who you are today the way that future you would have wanted to be treated?

____

____

4. Can you imagine a future you that is much kinder to themselves?

____

____

5. How do you lay the groundwork today to let future you feel loved?

____

____

"When you don't know what to do in a situation, ask yourself, 'What would the person I want to be do in this situation?' Then do that."

—Drew Dudley

When I asked a patient how this idea had helped, she said: *"I didn't always think that there would be a future me, let alone whether she would deserve a kinder future. I thought that the future would be hopeless, just an endless loop of hospitals and treatment programs. I never thought I would get to college. What really turned this around for me was applying to colleges. I realized that the future that I never thought would happen could actually happen. The next step was tacking the idea of being undeserving. Through the work we've done together, I've begun to challenge that. I now feel there is a part of me deserving of college, because that's what I have always dreamed about. Going to college would be a huge step in my journey, and I hope I get the chance to be future me at college."*

EXERCISE

Write down the experience of present you and all the negative self-talk and self-concepts that show up.

___

___

___

Next, imagine the person that is future you and all the things that you would want for them. Write down all the hopes and aspirations you have for that future version.

___

___

___

Remember, envisioning your future self is a powerful step toward positive change. By focusing on the hopes and aspirations for that future version, you set a foundation for growth and self-compassion. If you continue to practice self-criticism, self-loathing, and a negative self-view, there is no way to lay the groundwork for a more compassionate future self.

METAPHOR: If an apple tree is dying in poor soil today, enriching the soil with the things that the tree needs now will ensure that it is healthy and produces apples tomorrow. But here's the thing. Only you can guarantee that you tend to yourself. Other people may come and go into your life, and they may be helpful and compassionate, but the only person who is ever always going to be with you is you. You can make changes now that will nourish future you.

Why Connect with Your Future Self?

I want you to think about this: You know who needs you? Your future needs you. Your past doesn't. I am not saying that the past is irrelevant, but more that thinking about the past as if you could take care of it is much more difficult, if not impossible, than doing the things you need to now, for that future that absolutely needs YOU!

When you are suffering in the present, imagining a more self-compassionate self, even if you do not feel it now, can motivate you to do the things that you need to do now in order to be that future person. When you are hiking to the top of a high mountain, each step can feel difficult. The path is steep, and you are exhausted and every time you look up you feel no closer. But when the top is your goal, you need to take every step. You might slow down and rest, but never give up believing in a future self that has self-compassion and take the actions now. Let the vision of that future self be a magnet that pulls you there. This also helps you stay on task and overcome the difficult moments that are very likely to show up.

Your future self can also be a guide. If we continue with the hiking analogy, when you align your present moment to your future goal, you create a trail map for your journey toward the goal of self-compassion. It helps with choices; so for instance, will beating myself up now, or dating a person who devalues me, help me care for myself more in the future? Will taking the path that leads down the hill help me get to the top of the hill?

Connecting with your future self helps you overcome short-term distractions and short cuts. For instance, maybe dating the hurtful person lets you feel that at least you have someone in your life, and that after all you don't deserve anyone better. In a sense, this provides some short-term relief, however if you anchor yourself to a future self, you can imagine that person telling you not to date the hurtful person, even if in the short term it feels good. Imagine a future self, grateful to you for having made choices that they are now proud of. Ask yourself: "Will doing XYZ, get me closer to the person I want to be? Am I enhancing or perpetuating the person I want to become?"

Another idea is that if you can personify that future you, making that person a wiser you, the one that deeply knows you, future you can hold you accountable to your present action. They can encourage you to persist, and in this context, the future you can foster empathy for you now. Think of yourself when you were much younger, and maybe you were hurt by others, maybe you were demeaned, maybe you blamed yourself for everything. Can you have compassion for the you that suffered in the past? Can you imagine a future you having compassion for you now and also holding you accountable to making different choices?

The Psychology of Future Self

In psychology, there is a lot of future-self research that focuses on examining various ways and consequences of thinking about yourself in the future. Future self is part of a broader idea known as "Possible Selves." Of course, no one can know what the future is going to bring. We don't exactly know what tomorrow will look like, let alone the next year.

Stop reading for a second. I'll illustrate this in an exercise: take a slow in breath and slow out breath. Ready? Okay. Here is my question. "What is the next thought you are going to have?" We don't know because we can't know. So, if we can't even know the next thought we are going to have, how can we know tomorrow, or the next week, or so on.

ANALOGY: Let's imagine that your future self is a marathon runner while your present self is a couch potato. Although the future is uncertain, the habits you develop now will influence your likelihood of reaching that goal. If your present self commits to running daily, along with focusing on nutrition and sleep, you are more likely to develop into a future self that can complete the marathon. In contrast, if you remain inactive, eat poorly, and neglect rest, achieving that goal becomes much less likely.

However, there are many future possible selves. An academic self, an employed self, a family self, a relationship self, and so on. Each of those possible selves wants the ease of not hating themselves, and you can gift them that by doing things differently now. In the Psychology of the Future-Self studies, researchers explore how people perceive, relate to, and make decisions based on their concept of future selves. By focusing on future self and caring for that person in the way that you would want to be cared for, you are taking a step in the direction of eroding self-hatred. This idea is influenced by your present emotional attitudinal stance, and if you need to, you should go back and review this concept in Chapter 6. It doesn't happen overnight or all at once, but each time you invest in developing your future self by modifying one of your present behaviors, you move closer to becoming the person you wish to be.

Practicing a Degree of Self-Acceptance

> "You can't let your past define your future. Once you get that figured out, you begin to understand the joy of living in the present. And the present is full of tiny gifts that we can only see when we stop looking behind and ahead of us. Sometimes, these gifts land right at our feet. Sometimes, it's our feet that carry us toward them, running at full speed until our hearts nearly give out. Either way, never stop noticing them, and never stop wishing."
>
> —Cassia Leo

In CBT, the approach is the use of cognitive techniques to reappraise negative self-constructs such as self-hatred, in order to get rid of the constructs entirely. Many people find that this approach to self-hatred is an oversimplification of the symptom and is invalidating. An alternative is that of self-acceptance where self-compassion practices include ones where you can learn to accept your suffering.

EXERCISE

Break down your suffering into the following steps:

1. My suffering was caused. Write down the causes.

   ____

   ____

   ____

2. I recognize that I never chose to suffer and that it was never my goal to suffer.
3. I recognize that my suffering – which I did not cause – does not mean that I am a bad person.
4. I recognize that my suffering does not mean that I deserve to be hated.
5. I recognize that my suffering is not the same as self-hatred, but that self-hatred only makes my suffering worse.
6. I recognize that if I can accept that there have been hurtful things that happened to me and then recognize that these hurtful things have caused me to have negative thoughts about myself, that I can also appreciate the wonderful things in my life, and that hurtful and wonderful can coexist.

Doing Something You Love

> "You are not what you've done. You are what you keep doing."
>
> —Jack Butcher

I asked my patient collaborators whether there had been any extended periods of time that there had been relief from self-loathing and gained some interesting insight. Here's what one said:

> *"The only time I think it ever shifted was when I took a gap year in college. I went to work in Maine. Self-loathing went down for*

two reasons: I think partly because I was so busy doing something that made me really happy, and partly because I felt a sense of accomplishment and that I was good at something, which I legitimately had never felt to that degree before. But I definitely still noticed the self-loathing if I stopped to think about it. I don't think there were many days when the self-loathing was completely gone. Even though it was 'quieter' it was still very much there. When it did show up it was whether I was worried about if my boss hated me or if I had done something wrong or that I didn't actually know what I was doing and wasn't qualified for my job at all. Doing something you love and that you are good at helps, but the thoughts tend to creep in."

EXERCISE

Write down some of the things that you truly love doing.

____

____

____

____

____

Next, reflect on whether you actually do them. Commit to do the things that make you happier on a regular basis.

Noticing the Moments When the Feeling Changes

A few patients have told me that my repeated asking them about the topic and especially the focus on when it was strongest or least impactful was helpful. One patient said that it went from her thinking that it was there all the time to noticing that in fact it did change: *"For me, self-hatred is most prevalent under these circumstances: When my parents fight, when they argue about money, when my academic grades are being compared to my brother's grades, when I'm alone with my thoughts, and when I stand in front of a mirror. Self-hatred has much less of an impact in these circumstances: reading, watching a documentary about something I'm interested in, watching sports, and sometimes when I'm talking to people I care about. I notice when I read or write my self-hatred lessens a little. I found it interesting that there was any shift at all."*

EXERCISE

Notice moments when self-hatred is strongest and when it is weakest. Are there specific activities, people, situations, or environments when self-hatred grows or lessens?

YOUR ANSWER:

____

____

____

____

____

Comparing Yourself to Historically Loathed People

Once you have answered the questions asked earlier, and if you recognize that you and self-hatred are not the same thing, then here are some steps.

EXERCISE

If you think that you are that terrible, imagine that there are levels of loathsomeness. Think about people who you would categorize as the best people in the world, and those you would consider the worst. Now, focus on the worst, recognizing that your list may be different from other people's and then using facts, identify the actions and qualities that made them the worst.

YOUR ANSWERS:

____

____

____

Here is one person's answer: *"For me, Hitler, Stalin, and Mussolini were bad. Also, Dahmer, Bundy, Bin Laden. They murdered innocent people; they all had malice, intent. Hitler, Stalin, and Mussolini were all dictators, who, by nature, are evil and power-hungry people willing to kill to protect their control. Dahmer and Bundy are bad people because they were serial killers, and they both were evil. Bundy's youngest known victim was a 12-year-old girl. Dahmer ate some of his victims. Bin Laden was bad because he was terrorist. He orchestrated the attacks on the Twin Towers, killing thousands."*

I asked her if she was as bad as the people she had identified.

> *"Well, no. I am not as bad at all. I haven't killed anyone, or eaten anyone or terrorized anyone," she said. "I have always seen myself as terrible, but compared to those people, I don't think I'm bad, at least not to that degree. I don't want to be thought of in the same category as those evil men. I have never done anything as bad as they have done. Perhaps 'not great' is a better term, because it's not as harsh as bad, and by that thought, there are other people who probably burden the world more than I do. Thinking of myself as a burden, similar to them is not fair to me."*

The next week I asked, "Given that those are terrible people, are there people in a lesser category that are maybe not as bad, but that you would nevertheless not want others to think of you as in the same group?"

She answered: *"Some of our current politicians (names withheld), Putin, Lukashenko, my least favorite hockey player (name withheld), and another hockey player (name withheld) are the next tier down from the serial murderers from last week. (Names-withheld politicians) are bad people, at least to me, because their political views are too extreme and ultra controversial.*

Putin and Lukashenko are bad people because they both abuse their power. Putin is killing thousands in Ukraine and Lukashenko heads the only country even remotely helping Putin. The sports person (name withheld) is a bad person because he can be a dirty player and publicly supported Putin and Russia in the war in Ukraine. Another hockey player (name withheld) is a bad person because he badly hurt my favorite player Tuukka Rask of the Boston Bruins. I would not want to be thought of in the same category of any of these guys, so once again using the term 'not great' instead of bad is more fitting as it's more neutral."

EXERCISE

Now, consider the worst of your own behaviors. Reflect on the ways that you see yourself as unworthy and loathsome. Do you belong in the category of terrible people?

Are there things that you contribute to those around you, that make the world a better place, in the way that the people in your evil category don't?

YOUR ANSWERS:

____

____

____

I was in a therapy session with a patient who was certain that she was one of the most despicable people on the planet. When I asked her to compare herself to historically terrible people, she admitted that objectively she was not as bad as they were. She also asked the following: "How do other people answer this? Are the answers similar to mine?"

"Yes," I answered.

"Has anyone pointed out that they are all men?!"

No one had, but it is interesting that most of the people who have done objectively cruel and hateful acts to others have been men. I then asked her what her objective criteria are for being a good or a bad person, and this is what she answered: *"I think the key difference between a 'good' and a 'bad' person is the intention behind their actions. 'Good' people intend to positively impact people's lives, and when their impact and intentions don't align, they reassess what went wrong and commit to changing their behavior to align impact with intention. 'Bad' people intend to hurt others and do not feel remorse for their actions; they do not respect other people's humanity and continue hurting people even after seeing their negative impact on others, and I get it. Yes, if I use those criteria, I am not a bad person."*

EXERCISE

What is your objective definition of a good or bad person? Once you have answered that, do you meet the criteria for being an objectively bad person?

____

____

____

Identifying with the Qualities You Admire in People You Admire

> "She never felt sorry for herself, and that was something I decided I admired most in people."
>
> —Jeannette Walls

Even the most self-hating person, when they reflect truly on themselves, recognizes that they have some positive qualities. These include kindness, a sense of humor, being artistic, being curious, loyalty, being compassionate, and many others. The problem, however, is that often people who have these qualities, if they hate themselves, do not see these qualities as in any way reducing or impacting their level of self-loathing.

And yet, if I ask people to name people they admire, they are able to do so. If I then ask them to identify qualities about those people, they are able to do so. If I ask them whether they admire those people because of those qualities, the answer is almost always a resounding "yes." If I then ask my patients whether they themselves possess any of the qualities they admire in the people they admire, when they are honest with themselves, the answer again is almost always "yes." And so this then poses a conundrum. If you admire qualities in people you admire, and you yourself have those qualities, then how can you not admire at least that part of you?

EXERCISE

Now, consider qualities that you admire in people you admire. Reflect on whether you have some of those qualities. For instance, if someone you admire is compassionate and you find compassion to be an admirable quality, are you also compassionate and can you admire that in yourself? There may be qualities that you aspire to have in yourself. Are there things that you can do to develop those qualities?

YOUR ANSWERS:

____

____

____

Dismissing the Bullies and Tormentors of Your Past

> "One's dignity may be assaulted, vandalized and cruelly mocked, but it can never be taken away unless it is surrendered."
>
> —Michael J. Fox

A 20-year-old shared his idea: *"My parents sent me to a private boy's school in 5th grade, and it was very sports oriented, but I liked the arts. My self-hatred started when I got bullied for liking dance and music, and I used to go home every day and cry and felt that there was something really wrong with me. Why didn't I like football and basketball? They called me all kinds of names and even when I left after three years, all I could hear was their taunts and their jeers. I even turned that into a song:*

And then when I left
After three painful years
The memories I have
Are their taunts and their jeers.

So now, after we started talking about this, I realize that they are in my head and they are not in my life, but if I keep them in my head, I am allowing them to continue to bully me, so I fight back and kick them out:

You've lived in my head
And caused terrible pain,
But here's the thing boys
Get the fuCK out my brain

Yet, I didn't realize how much damage I was doing to myself by living as if they were still there. When I fight back, I feel a little victory and proud of myself, and I admire the me that fights back."

This reflection powerfully illustrates the idea of minimizing the amount of time that past negative experiences occupy space in your mind. By acknowledging that the taunts and jeers from your past are no longer part of your present reality and choosing to actively "kick them out" of your mental space, you reclaim your sense of self and assert dominion over your experience. It's important to recognize that these past experiences can only continue to hurt you if you treat them as if they were happening in the present moment. Each time you confront and reject these internalized voices, you are making space for a more positive and empowered version of yourself. This process of fighting back and celebrating small victories is a vital step in freeing yourself from the hold of past negativity and moving toward a healthier, more self-affirming future. You will read many versions of this idea throughout the book. Your task is to open yourself to the possibility that this concept is true and then to act as if it is. And if you think about it, you opened yourself up to the idea that self-hatred is true, what about the alternative?

EXERCISE

Who are your tormentors? Are they still around today? If not, how long ago did they leave? Do you still carry their damaging words? What were those words?

____

____

____

Realizing That Self-Hatred Was Learned

After having worked on self-hatred, here are the reflections of one patient: *"The idea that you are essentially taught to hate yourself is interesting, because this means that you can learn to love yourself. Also, the idea that some of the difficult moments in your life are necessary for growth is also a new way of thinking, rather than thinking that they are a reflection of how flawed I am. Then, and although it is still hard to wrap my mind around at times, the idea that we're all equal, is important, because I automatically assumed that other people's opinions about the world and me were more important than my opinions about the world and me. Next, I think that recognizing that I have a lot going for me, is important. I mean everyone has things going for them. I just thought that others' 'things' were more relevant, significant, and purposeful than mine.*

"It was also useful for me to think of self-hatred as an illogical conclusion, even though the logic behind the reasons why it develops makes sense. Also, when it was said that parents constantly hovering inadvertently teach their child that they cannot do things themselves, it surprised me because my mother constantly hovers. Finally, the idea that maybe they thought I am a burden, is simply a thought and not shared by others is actually quite liberating. I am still skeptical, but I continue to be willing to challenge that."

It's clear that these reflections highlight significant shifts in understanding and perspective. Recognizing that self-hatred is learned and not an intrinsic part of who you are opens the door to the possibility of self-kindness and acceptance. Seeing that many of life's challenges can be sources of growth rather than signs of some persistent and enduring personal flaw, reframes past experiences in a more constructive light. Further, that your knowledge of you, and your opinions about your place in the world, is as valid, if not more valid, than anyone else's, and certainly more valid than those who taught you that you were of little worth.

EXERCISE

Can you see that self-hatred was learned? How did you learn to hate yourself? What were the early lessons and who taught you?

____

____

____

Striving for Independence

Many people who struggle with self-hatred feel that they have very little dominion over their lives. It feels as if they are pushed into things or, that others are doing things for them, whether they want to or not. One patient told me: *"My parents were always telling me what to do. They didn't mean to be mean or anything, but I just could never do things on my own, and it reinforced how flawed I was compared to my friends and siblings."*

Here is the reflection of the impact of independent striving on the experience of self-loathing: *"My main achievement, and really first in a while, and the one that helped reduce self-loathing, was getting into college. The reason is because it was something I'd been striving for. All along the way, I told myself there was no way I could get into college, and in my darkest moments, would I even make it that far. I think, however, that my persistence in working for admission to college implied there was some part of me that believed it was possible to get myself to college. Getting accepted brought that part to the limelight. Instead of thinking that it was because of something my parents had done, I knew that I had done it. It was my striving and my purpose. For the first time, I had indisputable evidence that I had self-compassion, and even though a small part of me, I listened to it and it got me what I wanted."*

Claiming a sense of agency and independence plays a crucial role in overcoming self-hatred. The journey of striving toward your personal goals serves as a powerful affirmation of your capabilities. Your achievements not only highlight your own efforts and determination but also counter the internalized beliefs of inadequacy that have been fostered by external influences.

EXERCISE

You may have your own independent living ideas that would help you feel more autonomous over your life. My independence goals are:

____

____

____

Completing a List of Pros and Cons

DBT uses pros and cons as a skill to use in situations where decisions need to be made. In some ways, it is very similar to traditional pros and cons lists, however the skill in DBT has an important distinction. In DBT it is not only the pros and cons of doing something, but also includes the pros and cons of not doing something.

Once you have made your list, the next task is to circle the items in the list that are consistent with your wise-minded long-term goals. It is not simply the total number of items in any given column. For example, let's say that you had a test you had to take, and that you felt prepared for. You were out the night before, and you're exhausted and don't want to get out of bed. You might decide that there are so many pros to staying in bed. It's warm in your bed, you are still tired, you'll feel more rested if you wake up in a few hours, and so on. The con of staying in your bed is that you will get an incomplete in your transcript. So perhaps the list of staying in bed is much longer than that of getting up and taking the test, but the long-term consequence of not taking the test is much more significant than the short-term benefit of staying in bed.

If you accept, and by now I hope that you do accept, that self-hatred is learned and that it can change, then here is how the pros and cons skill would work.

	PROS	CONS
Tackling self-hatred		
Not tackling self-hatred		

	PROS	CONS
Being kind to yourself		
Not being kind to yourself		

The goal here is to look at the issue from all sides, by reviewing the pros and cons of each action and to decide what you are going to do going forward.

Focusing on the Wrong Side of Storytelling Versus the Right Side of Storytelling

> "Victim vs. Hero: When will you move from being the victim of your story to the hero? The moment you assume responsibility for your choices moving forward is the moment you recover and receive what you've been after."
>
> —Richie Norton

This is another wonderful idea shared by a deeply insightful patient. She is a prolific writer, and she had started to review some of her old writing and reflected on a piece of writing based on a hurtful interaction more than two-and-a-half years ago, when the idea struck her that at times there are ways that she tells stories that are not at all helpful to her, and that perhaps, without changing what happened, that there may be more useful ways to tell the same stories.

The wrong side of storytelling

September 2021

"My words don't fucking matter. I should just shut up. Everyone just thinks I'm complaining and externalizing. They don't listen to me and that is not going to change now. Just discharge me home and let me die. I am just an inconvenience to people, clearly. I don't know why I talk or why I try to get people to listen when the outcome is always the same. I thought maybe I deserved better treatment than how my therapist spoke to me, but I guess not. He is so clearly done being nice to me. I'm a piece of shit Borderline that is just angry and attacking. Well then why should I stay alive anyway? It doesn't matter what happens to me. People would get over it. I am boring and difficult to have around anyway."

She reread her writing and considered whether there was another way to review the event, and here is how she saw it recently.

The right side of storytelling

February 2, 2024

"Words wield so much power. A short paragraph from the archives has left me speechless, searching for which words could cradle a broken heart and mend a death wish. I can't find them. I feel helpless and I can't quite place why. She doesn't need saving. Not anymore. She only exists in the sense that I'm still here and in an additional sense that I am a firm believer of everything existing at once. But beyond this, she doesn't need my saving. Yet, my heart breaks for her – and it breaks for every soul that has had similar words. And maybe that's just it. Maybe, I see a little piece of myself in that paragraph but more than anything, I see anyone who has wished upon hopeless stars for their story's ending. One too many ugly stories we are told, and we wish to give up the rights to our story entirely. I read this paragraph, and this doesn't

feel like a story I wrote at all, yet I feel connected to the little girl that wrote endearing stories about magical mirrors and muddy buddies. I wonder why, but I answer my own curiosities as I often do through my writing. Despite being beyond alone with pieces of paper, I wrote that paragraph with the help of various co-authors. We aren't born hating ourselves. We aren't born missing the will to live. God didn't forget something. We are all here for something. I might have a million questions I will die with, and I might question the concept of purpose frequently, but at my core, I believe in it. We are all born storytellers, though stories we have our own unique languages for. We are all born with the unexplainable urge to tell stories, as living and storytelling are synonymous in my eyes. Many of us love ourselves up until we don't. Like self-love has an expiration date that depends solely on the environments that shape us. Maybe it doesn't happen all at once. Maybe we learn to hate ourselves in increments until it is all consuming. Maybe it feels near impossible to earn back the rights to your story when all you know is to look to others for their input. There are so many maybes, but I certainly can't be convinced that we are born hating ourselves. We are shaped for self-hatred through the stories we are told."

This patient demonstrates a profound shift in her perspective. Initially, her narrative was clouded by self-loathing and despair. Then, as she revisited and reframed her experience, she found a more compassionate and hopeful narrative. This transformation underscores the importance of how we tell our own stories. While the past cannot be changed, we can choose to reframe our experiences in ways that create a better environment for healing and self-acceptance. There is always room for growth and renewal in the stories we tell ourselves. This does not mean lying to yourself. If you were maltreated or abused, those things did happen. The reframing isn't in changing the truth. It is in changing its enduring effects, and making them less enduring.

EXERCISE

Reflect on an event or series of events that got you to believe that you were worthless. How do you tell that story? Does your answer lift you up? Is it helpful, or does it dig you further into a pit of false narrative? Now consider the same events and see them through a different lens, one where others, especially the hurtful people, DO NOT determine your worth, where you can see worth despite everything that has happened to you.

YOUR ANSWER:

1. The wrong side of storytelling.

2. The right side of storytelling.

Accepting the Current Moment

> "Acceptance doesn't mean you agree with, condone, or give up. It simply means you stop fighting reality."
>
> —Dan Millman

A former patient who had overcome self-loathing told me that accepting the current moment had been an important part of healing. *"My sister called me fat and ugly when I was young and my parents told me to let it be, that my sister was just teasing me. In kindergarten and elementary school, the kids were mean to me, and then by middle school, I let any boy do anything to me, because everyone told me that I would never amount to anything. Once I started to practice that maybe what they had said wasn't true, and as I started to practice acceptance of this moment, I realized that if all I did was ruminate about the past, all that I was doing was turning this moment into yesterday. But yesterday and all the horrible things that people did has gone. If all I did was spend time repeating what happened yesterday, in effect, I was making yesterday last forever."*

Wise words indeed: Holding onto past hurts can trap us in a perpetual state of suffering, distorting our ability to fully engage with the present. By choosing to accept and focus on the current moment, she began to break free from the cycle of self-hatred perpetuated by past events. It is another reminder that while you cannot change the past, you have the power to shape your experience today and move toward a more hopeful and self-caring future.

EXERCISE

What are the things that you have in the moment that you can be grateful for? Write them down whether big or small.

____

____

____

____

Practicing Core Self-Compassion

> "If all the world hated you and believed you wicked, while your own conscience approved of you and absolved you from guilt, you would not be without friends."
>
> —*Jane Eyre* by Charlotte Brontë

One patient told me that he outwardly practiced self-compassion, but not at an authentic level. He called it "surface-level," and these were his reflections: *"I think the difference between surface-level vs core self-compassion is the intention behind the actions I take. I see surface-level self-compassion as performing acts of self-care without connecting to self-respect or self-love. I can go through the motions of showering, resting, or going to therapy without doing the deeper work of nurturing self-esteem and truly accepting that I deserve care and love. Core self-compassion involves intentionally challenging my negative core beliefs and embracing the fact that, despite how I feel toward myself, I deserve the same compassion and dignity that others do."*

This can clearly be challenging for many, but perhaps the practice here is to do self-care and add the element of intentionally recognizing that it is compassionate to care for the self. And then, by recognizing that this is true for acts such as showering, eating, and going to therapy, then expanding the practice to other elements of your life.

EXERCISE

Think about some things that you do for yourself that show that you care about yourself. Perhaps your appearance, your compassion for others, or your dedication at work.

The ways in which I take care of myself, honor my values, and stick to my long-term goals are:

____

____

____

Now do the same exercise, and say: "and by doing these things, I am showing myself a little bit of self-compassion."

Another patient had a different take on her practice of core self-compassion. After we had started to tackle self-hatred directly, she noticed a shift that she termed "glimmers of self-compassion." I asked her to answer the following questions:

1. When do you notice the glimmers?
2. How can you start to believe that they are valid?
3. How do they begin to shift your self-hatred?
4. What can you continue to do to expand on seeing yourself in a more caring light?

> *"I have had a lot of glimmers of self-compassion in the last few days. Earlier this week, my family session at first felt like it really gave me a setback in terms of self-compassion. They reminded me of all the ways in which I had felt so bad about myself as a child, but the more I have processed it, the more I've felt myself be open to self-compassion. Having compassion towards my parents is helping me have more compassion towards myself because accepting that they did not know any better than they did, and then with the information that they had, that they did the best that they*

could, given their limitations, means that there was absolutely nothing I could've done to change the situation. I did the best I could, and there is nothing I could've done better to change the situation. And even if I could've, it's okay that I didn't because I was just a kid and creating a perfect childhood and reality was not my job. It's also a bit of a devastating phenomenon though because I put so much effort into fixing the situation, and I now realize that it was a futile effort and I put myself through all that pressure for nothing. I feel a lot of grief around this, but I'm also starting to feel compassion for a child that tried so hard to be perfect and who experienced so much pain around it. I have carried a lot of the baggage of that into my adult life. I think my next step will be to try and give the adult me who carries that baggage the same compassion and respect that I am working on giving to that confused and scared kid. I'm not completely sure how to do that, but I had a breakthrough about it during art therapy today and I'm working on a series about self-compassion and identity, so I'm going to continue to pursue that avenue of exploration, as well as talking about it in regular therapy sessions."

Self-compassion need not be some big act of self-love. These two people did it differently. The first recognized the act of self-care as compassion to the self. The second had compassion for parents who were ignorant of their impact, and compassion for a little girl who did not know what else to do. Both approaches highlight that self-compassion can come about in small, meaningful ways. Whether through nurturing yourself or understanding past influences or both, you can get on the path to healing from self-hatred.

Being Honest with Myself About the Value of the Work I Do

"Your self-worth grows when you fight for something you love."
—Maxime Lagacé

Often, people with core self-loathing reflect on the ways in which they are a burden to the world and don't, or won't, accept that their efforts have meaning and value to others. I have worked with teachers, nurses, doctors, and many people in the service profession who do incredible work, and who are valued for who they are, and yet won't see it, feeling that it is a mask. Yet the students and people they serve value them. I asked a patient to reflect on the ways in which she contributed, and to do so without editorializing, editing, or qualifying her reflection. This was her answer: *"One practice that helps me to erode feelings of self-hatred is my academic work. One of the primary thoughts that I have surrounding my self-hatred is that I do not add value to the world or that I am not capable of doing anything meaningful. I know objectively that the research I do contributes to the field and provides information that helps people. I often try to discredit this, but it is hard to do without blatantly denying the facts."*

By reflecting on your contributions, and doing so without self-criticism, you can start to recognize aspects of you that have value and impact, and when you see this, you recognize that no one with value and impact deserves to be treated with hatred, and you see that you can embrace these qualities within you.

Write down the ways in which the things that you do truly matter to other people:

____

____

____

Talking About It in Therapy

This is somewhat similar to the first one discussed: not being asked about it. In this one, you take more control of bringing it up. In recent years, I have asked therapist colleagues to start asking about self-hatred in their patients, especially as a part of their initial assessment. If self-hatred is not there, then no need to tackle it, but if it is, patients find it helpful. On the unit I work, therapists have started to talk to their patients about it, and it seems to be helping.

One patient reflected:

> *"Another thing that helps me to erode feelings of self-hatred is talking about it in therapy. I find it particularly helpful when the therapist questions my thoughts in a way that directly challenges what I'm saying in a way that is objectively/factually hard to argue against. My therapist often points out when I say things that contradict each other (for example, saying that I do not add value and then later saying I'm proud of work that I've done). This helps me to see that I do have positive beliefs about myself, even if I don't always acknowledge them."*

ACTION ITEM: Openly discuss it in therapy. As in an earlier exercise, this has to be intentional. In other words, don't hope that it comes up organically; instead, go to therapy with the intention of saying: "There is something I want to talk about today, and that is my self-hatred."

Checking the Facts

DBT has a skill known as "Check the Facts." It is most often used to help people manage their response to a situation by examining the factual evidence supporting their thoughts, feelings, beliefs and assumptions. The idea is to help people differentiate facts from interpretations, assumptions, or judgments, all of which can often be distorted by strong emotions. Although facts can cause us distress – for instance if you receive a failing grade on a test, you might be in distress – it can also be the interpretation, and then believing the interpretation that can cause even more distress. "I failed the test and so I will always be a failure." When it comes to self-hatred, some patients have told me that checking the facts has been helpful. For instance, the belief that everyone hates the person or that others would be relieved if they weren't around. I have had patients call others up to make sure that this is factually true, and of course, in no cases is it true. This approach does not work for everyone, because the counterargument is that "no one is going to tell me they hate me or that I am a burden. That would just be mean and the people who care about me are not mean." It's hard to argue against this when someone believes that they are so terrible; however, there are some for whom the approach helps somewhat.

How to Check the Facts About Self-Hatred

You can use this skill when you've had a spike in self-hatred.

1. (a) What is the event prompting the spike in self-hatred?

   (b) Describe the facts that you observed through your senses.

   (c) If you notice a judgment, an assumption, or a black and white thought, label those experiences as those experiences. Remember that judgments and assumptions are not facts.

   ____

   ____

   ____

2. Ask yourself: What are my interpretations of the events that prompted the spike in my self-hatred? For instance, say a friend did not return your call. Is your interpretation that they hate you? Are there other interpretations? Could you call them and ask? Remember that interpretations are not facts.

   ____

   ____

   ____

3. Ask yourself: How is it that I so quickly went to my interpretation? Do I benefit from having such a catastrophic thought? What if I took a neutral or even benign interpretation?

   ____

   ____

   ____

4. Finally: Given the facts that I have, do my interpretations and conclusions fit the facts?

____

____

____

A patient who was working on self-hatred told me that she had noticed a small reduction in the experience, and I asked her what had helped. Here's what she said: *"My self-hatred was always at a 100, and I went from a 100 to a 90 by defining what it means to be a 'good' versus 'bad' person and checking the facts to see if my actions actually aligned with my definitions. I also worked on reframing my ADLs (activities of daily living such as showering) as acts of self-respect, and in so doing to start to form a more neutral relationship with them. Additionally, I practiced radical acceptance surrounding the fact that I had to practice affirming my self-worth before I felt like I was ready for it or deserving of it."*

"That's great," I said, "so how do you go from a 90 to an 80?"

> *"I think going from a 90 to an 80 entails continuing to implement the strategies (checking the facts and radical acceptance) and exploring how to challenge the underlying causes of the self-hatred. I don't think there is a trick or shortcut to achieving self-compassion; I think it's mostly a process of repetition and practice that slowly rewires your brain to be more compassionate."*

I asked if she could dig deeper into how she used the skills and here are her responses:

a. How I use Check the Facts: *"I objectively described the facts of the situation, and reflected on whether the facts aligned with the actions/intents/characteristics that I identified as being associated with being a 'bad' person. By sticking to the objective facts and not my subjective interpretations of the facts, I was able to determine whether*

I actually did something that made me a 'bad' person, or if I had just felt like I did."

b. Defining "bad person" traits versus other: *"I found defining what makes a person 'good' or 'bad' to be helpful because it helped me check the facts and realize a lot of my self-hatred was grounded in my opinion of myself, rather than the actual facts. It also made me realize that the intention behind actions is the biggest difference between a 'good' and 'bad' person, which helped me realize that I'm not a actually a bad person."*

c. Seeing acts of self-care as self-respect: *"Seeing acts of self-care as self-respect has helped me develop a more neutral relationship with myself, which I see as the first step toward developing a kinder relationship to myself. In my personal experience, self-hatred has created a willfulness towards even considering self-compassion as something I can do. While it may seem like a matter of semantics to say something I do without much thought is self-compassion, the subtle shift helps challenge the willfulness and work towards self-compassion."*

The journey toward self-compassion is not linear, and it certainly does not happen overnight. However, as the patient's experiences illustrates, integrating practices like "Check the Facts" can chip away at the core construct of self-hatred. By distinguishing between facts and interpretations as well as recognizing the ways that you care for yourself, you begin to dismantle the false narratives that fuel your self-hatred. The practice of reframing activities of daily living as acts of self-respect and self-care and being clearer when using the labels of "good" versus "bad," you build the lens of discernment that provides a more accurate portrayal of who you are.

Tackling the Fear of Getting Better

Some patients have told me that they are afraid to get better. They tell me that they have been ill for so long and have had so much help along the way that they don't know what better feels like. They also fear taking responsibility for their own lives. *"My illness is all I know. It is my normal, and when I have moments of joy, they scare me because I think that they will go away. Feeling good makes me anxious, and to be honest, feeling bad makes me feel 'good' in that it is more comfortable and more familiar."*

One patient who was recovering from anorexia, a condition that for her was tied closely to her self-hatred, shared the following insights as to the struggle of her recovery and her getting better.

I asked her: As you recover from anorexia:

1. What does recovery body do to shame?

My weight-restored body elicits a lot of shame because I hate the way it looks and how it feels to exist in it. I feel like I looked better and more attractive when I was in my sick body, and I definitely mourn its loss, even though I logically know it wasn't healthy for me. Getting better scares me. My fear of others judging me negatively for how I look (that I'm ugly, lazy, gluttonous, etc.), along with my self-judgment of the same causes me to feel intensely ashamed of my body. My shame manifests as body avoidance and isolation, preventing me from engaging in platonic, familial, and romantic relationships.

2. What does the increase in shame do to your existing self-hatred?

"The increased shame around my body feeds into self-hatred because, in my mind, shame surrounding my body immediately morphs into shame surrounding myself as a whole, which then feeds into generalized self-hatred. Since my body feels so tied to my identity, hating my body causes me to hate myself, and both feed into each other in a vicious cycle. My self-hatred has gotten worse since weight-restoring, and I know I will need to work even harder to combat my self-hatred moving forward while maintaining my healthy weight."

3. Does acceptance feel too enduring?

"Accepting my weight-restored body feels daunting and impossible because existing in my body in the current moment is already overwhelming and difficult. Even the thought of staying in my body long-term evokes distress and intensifies urges to engage in ED

behaviors. I also fear that if I accept my weight-restored body forever, I will be an ugly, lazy, gluttonous person forever, and I fear the negative ramifications that would have on my self-image and my relationships with others."

4. What happens if you shift acceptance of everything that could happen to acceptance of just this moment?

   "Accepting my weight-restored body just in this current moment is still incredibly difficult, but less daunting than accepting my body for the rest of my life because it narrows down the time period to the present moment. Since I can actually control the present, it feels more achievable and tangible than trying to embark on the seemingly insurmountable challenge of accepting my healthy body forever, and in this context, the fear I have about getting better lessens."

EXERCISE

Do you fear getting better? What does this look like? What are the things in your life that you will no longer have if you are better? Are there ways to manage this fear so that you don't lose everything all at once? What are the things you might gain?

The journey of addressing self-hatred and replacing it with a more accurate and compassionate version of who you are is a complex and deeply personal one. On this journey you will grapple with long-standing fears and habits that have shaped your sense of who you are. The fear of getting better, as shared by many, underscores the comfort found in the familiar, even when that familiarity is steeped in pain and illness. The recovery process can also bring to light the intertwined nature of physical and emotional healing.

By examining the reflections of those in recovery, or those who have recovered, you see the importance of integrating therapeutic strategies such as "Check the Facts," which helps in separating fact from interpretation and assumption. This, and many of the other ideas, is an integral part of the road map to seeing yourself in a kinder and more complete way.

These shared experiences highlight the incremental nature of progress. Accepting the present moment, rather than the daunting prospect of a lifetime, can make the process of healing feel more manageable. Each small step, whether it's recognizing a positive trait or reinterpreting a negative belief, contributes to a more compassionate self-view.

Be patient. Say it to yourself: "I must be patient." Be persistent. Say to yourself: "I have to push on every day." Be willing. Say to yourself: "I am willing to challenge the distortions I was taught." In as much as the stories you have read serve as a testament to the resilience of the human spirit and the transformative power of compassion, your story can, too.

In the next chapter, I'll review other promising ideas and treatments that could be useful in overcoming self-hatred.

Chapter 15

Alternative Treatment Ideas

The following ideas are ones that have the theoretical potential to help. I include them because there are enough individual case reports of recovery. Also, because there is some science that supports their inclusion, and so they merit further exploration.

Psychedelics

> "Psilocybin can help us break down the barriers between ourselves and others and foster a sense of empathy and compassion."
>
> —Katherine MacLean

I was at a conference and was approached by a therapist who knew of my interest in tacking self-loathing. He told me that he had BPD and that he had struggled with self-hatred for much of his life:

> *"Growing up, my family was not emotionally expressive and whenever I was upset, their main approach was to tell me to 'calm down.' After graduating from high school, I went to college on the West Coast, and to be honest, it was to study psychology. After completing freshman year, I decided to try to explain to my family what BPD was and what it was like to live with BPD. I told them about my intense and painful emotions and that more than anything I would have loved to have been able to calm down whenever I was upset. I told them that I understood why they had told me to calm down but that it had never been helpful because, even though they couldn't understand why I was so upset, their instructions made*

me feel terrible about myself, and that I felt broken for not being able to control my emotions. I also explained that it was always confusing to me why others didn't get as upset as I did, and that even when they did get upset, that they knew how to calm down, but that I didn't know how to. I knew that the others in my family didn't seem to get as worked up and that I thought that maybe it was because I had something seriously wrong with me, and that they were all okay. It was then that I started hating myself, hating the flawed individual I was. I was honest: 'My flaw is that I am so emotional and a burden to you all. I wish that I could just get rid of my emotions.' My parents listened carefully, and then my dad said: 'There is nothing wrong with you! All you need to do is to love yourself.' I knew that his intentions were well-meaning, but I felt more misunderstood than before."

All his interactions with other people, and even his self-reflections and judgments about self-hatred, were filtered through a voice that told him that he was irreparably flawed. He concluded that not only did he not like living with the constant thought that he was flawed, but that his emotionality, his irreparable flaw, made him such a burden, that suicide was the only solution. With that came a series of increasingly potentially lethal suicide attempts. *"But then something happened that changed how I saw myself and how I saw my place in the world,"* he said. *"One of my college roommates told me about psychedelics and how they had helped him. I started micro dosing. The first thing I noticed was that the focused voice of negativity suddenly no longer dominated my thinking. I had never experienced that before!"*

A friend of a friend: The daughter of a friend of a friend asked if she could talk to me. She knew that I worked with people who struggle with BPD and wanted to ask my opinion on psychedelics, and she shared the following experience:

"I struggle mostly with not liking myself very much. I feel that I am much too much for other people. Therapy has helped, but not a lot with this and none of my medications have ever helped.

A friend at college let me know about mushrooms. I am not a drug user; I mean not non-prescribed drugs but my friend's experience seemed amazing. Here's my experience:

Pre-micro dosing: *"Before micro dosing mushrooms, I used to feel extremely attached to my own ego and emotions within my human experience. I believe we have a soul that can travel across lifetimes, and a physical body that appears in the form of who we currently are. Often times I feel like because of my BPD, my soul and my physical, human self are constantly at odds. My deepest core desires to love others and be loved in a way that feels liberating conflicts with my body's extreme reactions to certain triggers or even stimuli. My body becomes entirely controlled by my very intense, human thoughts. It feels like someone else has taken control over my brain and I am just in the back seat, watching this other person destroy my sense of self and my life, and I don't feel very good about myself at all.*

Post-micro dosing: *"Micro dosing expands my awareness, which in turn opens my heart. When I take mushrooms, I have an out of body experience, where I feel that I can see myself from a birds-eye view, non-judgmentally. This perception of myself from a "birds-eye view" is not critical nor harsh, it is rational, wiser. It allows me to mindfully observe certain patterns within my life that are unhealthy or self-destructive, without being so deeply attached to my own negative emotions. There is a level of detachment I experience while micro dosing, a greater distance between myself and my ego. This expanded awareness and perception makes my heart feel more open; more open to feeling deeply whether the emotion is joyous or painful. And the opening of my heart over time creates more contentment, because I am able to accept myself and others despite whatever flaw there is.*

"It was only with the use of psychedelics that I was able to open to the idea that I could be worth it."

Cautionary Notes and Research

CAUTIONARY NOTE: At the time of this writing, there is no medication or psychedelic that treats self-hatred. There is no specific dose, or recommendation as to the level of psychedelic that would be helpful for self-loathing. I am neither endorsing nor rejecting the use of psychedelics and include this section because there is data that could support their use. Because the unrelenting suffering caused by self-hatred leads those who struggle with it to seriously contemplate, and at times act on, suicide, the research on psychedelics and their role in treating self-loathing has to be seriously considered. More and more therapists are being trained in psychedelic assisted psychotherapy, and this could offer a more immediate option, in conjunction with talk therapy, as a possible alternative idea.

ANOTHER WORD OF CAUTION: If you have bipolar disorder, you should know that some psychedelics are activating so there is the possibility that their use could trigger a manic episode. In a survey of 541 people with bipolar disorder (Morton et al. 2023), one-third of respondents described new or increasing symptoms after psilocybin trips, and these were mainly manic symptoms, difficulty sleeping and anxiety. In their study, they found that the side effects were of such concern that they needed to use the emergency department (fewer than 4%), and that all of the respondents, even those who experienced negative side effects, said that psilocybin use was more helpful than harmful.

With the two aforementioned accounts of dramatic changes in self-construct, I decided to do some research into how they might possibly reduce self-hatred. The therapist and the daughter of the friend of a friend appeared to be onto something.

Research: Making the Case

Here is the case for considering psychedelics based on our current understanding of brain function, and this section includes a lot of brain science and anatomy and reading it will help to understand why psychedelics may work.

The prefrontal cortex (PFC): The PFC is considered to be your "personality center" and is the part of the brain that makes you the you that you are. The PFC is where you process moment-to-moment information from your surroundings, compares the present-moment information to past experiences, which in turn causes you to react in some way. The PFC is also the part of the brain that allows you to make decisions and plan for the future.

The default mode network (DMN): The DMN is a network that connects different parts of the brain, including the PFC and is typically active when you are not focused on the outside world, meaning that it is active when you are daydreaming, ruminating, thinking about yourself, or thinking about others. It turns out that in people with depression, anxiety, post-traumatic stress disorder, attention deficit hyperactive disorder, schizophrenia, and obsessive-compulsive disorder, their DMN does not work as it is supposed to (Gattuso et al. 2023). It also turns out that in people with conditions such as depression, when they focused on negative images, their DMN became more active and stayed focused on negativity as compared to people without depression (Sheline et al. 2009).

When looking at the activity of the DMN in people with BPD, the researchers found a disruption in the DMN leading to difficulties in emotion regulation and processing their sense of self (Amiri et al. 2023). The authors proposed that psychotherapy may work through correcting the DMN connections, and that this correction is associated with positive changes in BPD emotional symptoms.

Putting It All Together

Psychedelics and the DMN: Because negative mind wandering and negative self-referential thinking are so active in conditions such as depression and BPD, anything that could reduce this negative activity in the DMN might be helpful in reducing the negative experience of self. It appears that psychedelics do just that. Micro dosing of psychedelics such as psilocybin – micro dosing refers to taking doses below the amount where you would hallucinate – has been shown to reduce mind wandering, and this correlates with a reduction in activity in the DMN. Users of psychedelic drugs often report that their sense of being a self, an "I" that is different from the rest of the world, and that separateness seems to evaporate or dissolve altogether. The point is that if you are stuck in a brain experience that is "I," "I," "I," all the time, and if the "I" is followed by statements like "don't like myself," "hate myself," or "am to blame for everything," then by breaking the centrality of the negative "I" you see that you are more than a concept and you begin to see yourself as much more than an awful person.

Further Reflections

I asked the person to tell me more about her experience and she continued: *"It's not some epiphany. I still have the voice that tells me that I am a terrible person. It just doesn't dominate any longer, and even when it lingers, I don't believe it like I used to. If I wanted to go down the well-worn path of self-loathing, I could easily do that. Sometimes, I'll even dwell in that thought for a few minutes, just to realize how much it has changed. What's changed is that it no longer controls my whole experience and that I no longer tolerate abusive behaviors from others. In the past I believed that I deserved abuse as punishment, but that's all gone. The one thing that is important is that if I stop micro dosing, the voice comes back stronger and stronger. I tried to quit once, but after a few weeks I was back to square one with self-loathing, so maybe it would be better to do it with therapy. Some people, OK my parents, tell me I shouldn't need it all the time. But my dad is on antidepressants every day, and my mom takes antianxiety pills all the time. I don't see those helping them as much as micro dosing helps me. And there is another thing. I am making friends again. I wondered why I had no friends, but all I used to do was to complain to people about how much I sucked and how much my life sucked. I stopped doing that and now people actually like me. When that negative self-loathing voice quietened down, I saw that the way people saw value in me was real. I have stopped doubting that I have worth, and micro dosing has helped me in ways that no other medication or therapy has. I definitely feel that maybe I could use some skills that could help in case it no longer works. Before I would not have believed that I could do something like self-compassion but now I am open to it."*

Wise words indeed; however, I want to reiterate the caution that there is no long-term research study on psychedelic medication for self-loathing. Taking a medication that could potentially cause psychedelic effects could worsen certain mental health conditions, and many unregulated hallucinogens are cut with other drugs. Remember too that not everyone's response will be the same, and so if it is a consideration there are now Psychedelic-Assisted Therapy Providers (PATP) who are trained in the administration of these substances.

Improving Your Heart Rate Variability (HRV)

The reason I include heart rate variability (HRV) is that many of the conditions tied to self-hatred are ones where people have low HRV. Further, research shows that as HRV improves, psychiatric distress symptoms reduce. In theory, if a person feels fewer symptoms of their disorder, their self-loathing will reduce. There is no research that proves this; however, the research on HRV and mental health is compelling.

HRV is a measure of the fluctuation in time between heart beats. It turns out that this period of time is not exactly the same between beats; however, these fluctuations are not something that you can measure by taking your pulse. Instead, you need a device such as an electrocardiogram (EKG) machine. What is interesting is that abnormal HRV can indicate current or future health problems, including cardiac conditions and mental health issues such as anxiety, depression, post traumatic stress disorder (PTSD), and borderline personality disorder (BPD).

In summary: Your heart is constantly beating and needs to do so in order to keep you alive. The rate at which it beats depends on what you're doing at the time. When you're resting, your heart beat is slower, and when you're active, or stressed or highly emotional, it beats faster. HRV is not about your heart rate. Instead HRV is the time between heart beats.

To explain it differently, imagine that you are driving down a road and there are 60 telephone poles along the road. Say that they are spaced 50 ft apart. In this case, the variation between poles is very low, meaning that they are all 50 ft apart. Now, say that on another road with 60 poles, they were spaced out differently. Some 20 ft apart, others 30 ft apart, and others 60 ft apart. The variation would be high. So even though both roads have 60 poles, the variability would be different. Two people may have the same number of beats per minute, one with low variability and one with high variability.

Your heart does not automatically know when to increase in speed or to stay at rest. It relies on information from the outside. Your heart does not know that a lion chasing you means that you need to get your heart rate up. Your heart relies on information from a part of your nervous system known as the autonomic nervous system. Your senses, meaning your sight, sound, smell, taste, and touch receive information and send it to your brain. Your brain then makes a decision about the situation and then sends a signal directly to your heart, telling it that it needs to speed up and work harder, in a situation where you are in danger or exercising. In the case of the charging lion, your eyesight would pick up that the lion was coming at you and you would hear its growling. That information would be rapidly turned into a chemical signal, sent along the autonomous nervous system, and it would tell your heart to beat faster.

Now, your autonomic nervous system is working all the time, even when you're asleep. It's divided into two main parts: the sympathetic nervous system and the parasympathetic nervous system.

The **sympathetic nervous system** is where the so-called "flight-or-fight" response comes from. In emergency situations, it controls increases in heart rate and blood pressure in order to prepare your body to act. In the case of the lion charging, it prepares you to run to the nearest tree, or if there is no tree, to stand your ground and fight.

The **parasympathetic nervous system** is the counterbalance to the sympathetic nervous system and is in charge of the relaxation response, especially after you've been in a flight-or-fight situation. It controls decreasing your heart rate and blood pressure, as well as other body functions, in particular when you need to relax. So, once you had been rescued from the lion, your parasympathetic nervous system would kick in and tell you that the danger is over and that you can relax.

So, you have one set of nerves telling your heart to beat faster under certain circumstances, and another set of nerves telling your heart to slow down. Here is where HRV comes in. In people who are mentally and physically healthy, their heart speeds up when it has to, and slows down when it needs to. In people with certain mental health conditions, the brain is constantly sending signals to the heart that there is something wrong, even when there isn't.

What this means is, for healthy people, the difference in heart rate between fight-flight situations and calm states is high. The heart can rapidly change to what the situation needs. For people with certain mental health conditions, their brains send signals to the heart that everything is a threat and dangerous, so, when they are in an actual fight-flight situation, their heart rate is high. But unfortunately, even when they are in a supposedly calm, and not dangerous situation, their brain continues to send danger signals, and so their heart rate remains high. This means that there is very little variation between danger states and calm states and so their HRV is low.

Other than certain cardiac and mental health conditions, aging is also something that causes a decline in HRV. In fact, HRV decreases significantly as people get older. In 20–25-year-olds the average HRV is in the 55–105 range, while in 60–65-year-olds the average is 25–45.

Here is another sobering concern: Multiple studies have shown that lower HRV is associated with a shorter lifespan, the risk of obesity, heart disease, inflammation, and lower immune response to viruses.

BOTTOM LINE: A high HRV is good and a low one is something you want to change.

HRV and Mental Health Conditions

HRV and PTSD: Many people reading this book will have been diagnosed with PTSD. PTSD is a psychiatric diagnosis that can develop in some people who have experienced or witnessed a traumatic event. According to the DSM (APA 2022): "The person was exposed to: death, threatened death, actual or threatened serious injury, or actual or threatened sexual violence, in the following way(s): Direct exposure. Witnessing the trauma. Learning that the trauma happened to a close relative or close friend."

HRV has been shown to be lower in people with PTSD. In a study that measured HRV in three different groups (Hauschildt et al. 2011): The first group were people who had experienced trauma, who then went on to develop PTSD, the second was a group who had experienced trauma who had not developed PTSD, and the third was a group of controls, meaning a group of people who had never experienced trauma, and therefore had not developed PTSD. The researchers found that people with PTSD had a lower HRV than the control group. Remember, lower HRV is unhealthy. Interestingly, the group who had experienced trauma but who had not developed PTSD did not have lower HRV.

What is important to know is that studies have shown that as people improve from PTSD, that their HRV also improves. For instance, in a study of veterans with PTSD, participants were randomly assigned to receive either HRV biofeedback plus treatment as usual (TAU) or just TAU (Tan et al. 2011). The results showed that HRV biofeedback significantly increased the HRV while their symptoms of PTSD reduced. For people who received non-specialized treatment, or TAU, there was no significant effect on either HRV or symptom reduction.

HRV and BPD: Similar to PTSD, studies have shown that people with BPD also have lower HRV (Back et al. 2022). In one study on BPD and HRV (Weise et al. 2020), the researchers showed that adolescents with BPD who had higher HRV at the start of DBT treatment, did better in terms of symptom reduction than those with lower HRV at the start of treatment. Further, as the patients improved, their HRV improved.

BOTTOM LINE: Low HRV is associated with symptomatic PTSD and BPD, and as a person improves from PTSD and BPD their HRV improves. The flipside of this is that improving HRV reduces PTSD and BPD symptoms. You may find this interesting, but what does this have to do with self-hatred? Read on!

Research on Improving Your HRV

Self-Compassion and HRV

Earlier we reviewed the practice of self-compassion. A study (Kim et al. 2020) looked at participants' responses when they faced disappointments such as rejection or failure. They examined the way the participants dealt with the disappointment and focused on whether they used self-criticism or self-reassurance to self-regulate. The researchers also looked at the participants' HRV. They found that those who practiced self-compassion had an increase in HRV. They also found that people who began the trial with lower resting HRV, and practiced self-compassion derived even more benefit as measured by even higher HRV and increased self-compassion. If you are up for practicing self-compassion to improve your HRV, here are the steps:

Step 1: Be honest with yourself and acknowledge that you are suffering.

Acknowledge that your default position is one of self-hatred and that it causes you to suffer. And likely, when you suffer, it is understandable that you don't want to examine it and feel the pain of the suffering. It is possible that you are using escape and avoidance strategies that help in the short run, but that in the long run cause you more suffering, behaviors like self-harm, drugs, alcohol, and dangerous relationships.

EXERCISE A: What are the behaviors I do to escape from the experience of self-hatred?

____

____

____

____

____

EXERCISE B: Identify someone you love. (NAME). Now imagine that they are asking you for help with emotional suffering. Would you recommend the behaviors you are doing in Exercise A as a way to deal with their pain? Y/N

Imagine you suggested self-harm, drugs, alcohol, or a dangerous sexual behavior. Would this be a caring response to give them?

EXERCISE C: What would you tell your loved one (NAME) if they were struggling? What words would you use?

____

____

____

Now replace their name with yours.

Step 2: Be kind, remembering that you are fundamentally kind, even if you don't fully believe it.

Many people with self-hatred don't believe that this will change. Practicing believing that they are kind can seem like an impossible task. And yet, many people with self-hatred do believe that they can act out of kindness toward others; and so, there is kindness inside of them.

EXERCISE A: Identify all of your self-critical statements.

____

____

____

EXERCISE B: Be there for yourself in the kind way you would be there for someone you care about. Replace the kind statements that you would use for other people with kind statements for yourself. For instance, if they screwed up, what would you say? Would you say, "I am here for you?" Or would you say, "you screwed up, you are a terrible person?" Replace your self-critical statements with kind, or at least kinder, statements.

Exercise C: Don't compare yourself to others. Some people with self-hatred compare themselves to others who appear to be worse off. Maybe others have much less money, a worse job, an abusive partner. Do you make statements like "I should not feel this way because, (NAME) has it worse off"? Remember that you do not know the lives of others and the only person you should be comparing yourself to is yourself. If you are working on self-hatred, acknowledge that you are doing so today. "Today, I am working harder on being kinder to myself. That is different than yesterday when I wasn't working on being kind to myself."

Breathwork and HRV

As I've mentioned throughout the book, many people with self-hatred find the practice of self-compassion to be difficult, if not impossible, to do. Earlier in the book I covered some of the comments from patients who told me why it was such a difficult thing to do. If you have difficulty practicing the earlier self-compassion exercises, research (Russell et al. 2017) shows that there are many other ways to improve HRV. One of the ways is through breathwork and one specific exercise is to slow the rate at which you breathe. The researchers showed that a slow, paced breath for as little as six minutes a day can improve your HRV.

EXERCISE

One effective way to practice this is to inhale slowly for say five to six seconds, to then hold your breath for four seconds, and then exhale slowly for seven or eight seconds. The goal is to breathe in deeply, into your belly, and then exhale through pursed lips. If you do this breath exercise, you'll be breathing at a rate of four to five breaths per minute.

Balanced Exercise and HRV

Regular exercise has many physical and mental health benefits, and many who read this book will have heard that they need to exercise. Exercise has the added benefit of improving your HRV. In a study that looked at the role of exercise and the relationship between HRV, acute stress, and perspective taking in a young female sample (Kähkönen et al. 2021), the researchers found that low HRV was associated with greater difficulty in perspective taking. They also found that those who exercised regularly had higher HRV and had improved perspective taking even under stressful situations. Their findings suggested a close link between physiological stress regulation and social cognition, and that exercise improved HRV, reduced stress, and improved social cognition.

Pleasant Memories and HRV

In a study (Gadeikis et al. 2017) where researchers looked at what happened to HRV when people focused on pleasant memories or thoughts (ones that induced positive moods) versus negative memories (ones that induced negative moods), they found that recollecting positive memories led to an improvement in HRV, whereas recollecting negative memories led to a reduction in HRV. A similar study (Kop et al. 2011) where the researchers examined the impact of inducing positive moods versus negative moods found that HRV improved during positive mood induction. I find these articles to validate my own experience. An exercise that I have done with some patients is to ask them to create a physical or virtual album with photos of the past events that made them happy and then to bring the album into session. The goal here is not to reject, deny, or forget the negative things that have happened to you, but instead to also focus on positive memories as a way to remember that there have been some wonderful events in your life.

EXERCISE

Find the photos that have captured the joyful moments in your life. Turn these into a joyful album of positive memories. Look over your album when you are feeling low.

Eye Movement Desensitization and Reprocessing (EMDR)

> "You have an internal critic, an internal drive that says, 'OK, you can do more.' Maybe that's what keeps you going. Maybe that's a demon. . . . Some people say, 'It's a muse.' No, it's not a muse!

It's a demon! DO IT YOU BASTARD!! HAHAHAHAHAHAHA!!! THE LITTLE DEMON!!"

—Robin Williams

Eye Movement Desensitization and Reprocessing (EMDR) is a type of psychotherapy used in people with trauma, anxiety, and other mental health disorders. It involves recalling a stressful event and "reprogramming" the memory using rapid eye movements. The goal is to change the way the memory is stored in the brain, which in turn reduces or even eliminates traumatic memories.

EMDR theory states that when you are traumatized, your brain stores the trauma memories in a way that doesn't allow you to accept the message that the danger is over. It tells you that the danger continues to be present and that this then leads you to have negative core beliefs and cognitions. These core beliefs have three characteristics; they are: negative, irrational, and self-referential. For instance, the child who believes "I did something wrong," can then start to believe "I am a bad person," and this thought can become deeply embedded into their personality structure, and the deeper it gets stuck, the harder it is to change. Many people who experience this type of trauma end up with enduring self-hatred.

If you believe that you are completely unlovable, that not even your parents loved you, that they rejected you, you might then come to the belief that you are a burden and that you should never have been born in the first place. Then later in life, even if you have kind or loving experiences, instead of seeing these as loving, the experience becomes connected to your early trauma experiences and memories and ends up reinforcing your negative beliefs, over and over again. For instance, if you experienced emotional or sexual trauma as a child, your body develops physical trauma reactions that can lead to an enduring sense of self-disgust and seeing yourself to blame for what happened. Then when there is a future intimate moment of tenderness and compassion, rather than seeing it as loving, your trauma-related body sensations remind you of the maltreatment, and then is repulsed by any genuine display of physical affection.

It is these cognitions where EMDR can help. During EMDR you pay attention, for short bursts of time, to emotionally difficult material while focusing on an external object. The best-known external focus is moving your eyes from side to side by tracking something that the therapist is holding, but therapists also use hand tapping or audio stimulation. The task is to focus on the painful memory and then identify the beliefs you have about yourself that were caused by, and connected to, that painful, often negative memory. As an example, say that as a kid you were frequently punished for having emotional outbursts, and this then led you to believe that you are a bad person, and a burden to your family.

During the EMDR session, you would formulate a positive belief that you would like to have about yourself; for example, "I am a compassionate and kind person." You would identify all the physical and emotional experiences associated with the memory and then, you would repeat the memory over and over, while focusing on the external object, until the point that the memory is no longer disturbing. The therapist then instructs you to replace the negative belief, with the new, positive belief. The theory behind the efficacy of EMDR is that in moving your attention from side to side, you bypass the part of the brain that has become stuck with the negative belief that was caused by the trauma. Over time, you begin to process the memory in a way that leads to a more peaceful experience and in so doing, long-held negative beliefs begin to change. Using the previous example where you were punished for being sensitive, through the EMDR process you come to realize that you were not to blame for what happened, that you are now safe in the world, that the punishment was a thing of the past, and that you are in control of your experience.

There are two interesting and important points to consider. On the one hand, many trials of EMDR exclude people who are suicidal and have made a suicide attempt in the past six months, and because people with core self-loathing can present with significant suicidal ideation, some practitioners might determine that they are not candidates for the treatment. On the other hand, a study that looked at EMDR in 97 people with personality disorders and without PTSD (Hafkemeijer et al. 2020), the researchers found that after three months, when compared with patients who had not received

EMDR, those who did the EMDR therapy showed significant and persistent improvements, and so EMDR may be a useful approach.

If EMDR therapy sounds interesting to you, websites such as https://www.emdria.org/find-an-emdr-therapist/ have lists of people who practice EMDR.

In the evolving landscape of mental health treatment, new scientific applications are being turned into therapeutic measures that could help people who are struggling with self-loathing. Some can help improve mood, offering a potential pathway to disrupt negative thought patterns and others improve emotional distress and reduce negative thinking, helping people reframe their self-perception. These innovative therapies are new ideas, ones that seem to be more holistic approaches for treating self-loathing by addressing both the psychological and physiological aspects of mental health. As research continues to expand, integrating these methods into other treatment protocols could offer new hope for those seeking to overcome deeply ingrained negative self-constructs, including self-hatred. In the next chapter, we'll review the experience of people who have overcome or have recognized the instability of the certainty of self-hatred as core.

Part 5

Finding Hope and Technology's Limits

Chapter 16

The Dawn of Hope

"Any person capable of angering you becomes your master; he can anger you only when you permit yourself to be disturbed by him."
—Epictetus, Stoic philosopher born into slavery

I would not have embarked on this quixotic journey without the remarkable stories of hope, told by those who have challenged the false narrative of self-hatred. The journey out of self-hatred is not a feel-good story. The path is difficult, but worth it in the end. Here are a few accounts of the trek our of self-hatred hell. They capture hope despite the many moments of struggle. They show how something that can feel so stuck can, in fact, change. Here are some reflections:

I Belong

"I was trying to get some deeply desperate needs met. I didn't truly believe that I was an attacking person, but because I was still becoming the stories I was told, I would add it to my pages and refer back to it for future episodes of self-loathing. That became my evidence for the ways in which I hated myself. This many people have disliked you. This many people hated you – and here's why. This many people made you feel small, so you must be small. This many people took your voice away; this is data to remain voiceless. My diagnosis and its symptoms were newer evidence in that they hadn't always had words to describe them. My illness hadn't always flourished, either. Now that it did and now that I had a

diagnosis with an entire bullshit story I could be reduced to, I had even more to work with.

"Vulnerable people take weaponized words at face value. They don't question what doesn't make sense, at least not out loud. They become things they never were. They acquire wishes that would relieve others of their faults and inadequacies in theory. If I was told I was attacking and if it were inferred that I was just being my symptoms, I'd lean right into it. I'd fulfill their prophecy because I, too, hated me. I, too, only saw an illness and failed to see a human. Behind closed doors they'd talk of the alleged self-fulfilling prophecy that is BPD. You're asking me to be different, to recover from my illness willingly but your idea of meeting me halfway was recreating my invalidating childhood environment that resulted in that illness. Ironies by the dozen and I live for them, now. I can see clearly now and here is what I see: I never really hated myself. I hated the stories I was told. God, I hated the stories I was told.

"There is, however, one part of that paragraph I still believe in: I have never belonged here. I take it back; I was right about more than one thing. They were never going to listen to me. That ultimately was the truth, but my perspective was distorted. My words would be twisted and manipulated and the moment that happens, you leave. You don't stick around waiting for some plot twist where one day, they listen. You unpack your baggage and this time, it just feels different. They get it now. No, you pack the baggage the moment you are abused for having unpacked it. They never got me, and they had been committed to never getting me. The same way stories were written for me, I wanted people and things to live up to my expectations and when they wouldn't, I wouldn't come to the conclusion that they weren't for me. I would give undeserved opportunities for people to be as good as I thought they should be in my head. I'd see them for what they were, but I'd want so desperately for them to be different, to be better. So, I'd stick around waiting on their character

development instead of investing in mine – and I was always disappointed in the end. With distorted vision, I only saw that I never belonged here. I didn't see belonging as something I could learn not to value much. I didn't see that feeling inherently different could have more perks than anything. Many things I hated about myself I have learned to value, and I'd even reserve the word love for some of those things.

"Tonight, I write a note that I store safely in my mind. I thank her for her wisdom because tonight, I learn. You never hated yourself; you only hated the stories you were told – and those stories you became. In becoming, I also believed and in believing, I learned to hate. Oh, look at my little words mattering. I never thought I'd see the day."

Choices

"Every day, I make choices. Of course, I did not choose the things that happened to me, but I learned to choose how I react. In fact, choosing is the only real option I have. Choosing how I react: CHOICE.

"Even though I have been hurt by the people who were supposed to love me, and when they hurt me because of the choices they made, ones that cause me pain, I can let it go. Choosing to let it go: CHOICE.

"And then there was marijuana. It blissfully lifted me out of suffering by numbing me out. Sure, being high all the time affected my relationships and my work. Choosing to stop getting wasted: CHOICE.

"I disgusted myself with my behaviors, and for a long time I continued to do them, even though I knew that I was crossing my values and debasing myself. I did nothing about my behavior. I avoided thinking about my responsibility in my actions and how I felt: Choosing to address these in therapy: CHOICE.

"Today I am on the path to overcoming the self-hatred I learned, and that is a CHOICE!"

I Am Okay

"The bullying by the mean girls started when I was in the 5th grade. I didn't know that they were mean at the time, only that the things that they did and said were very hurtful. My parents were going through a divorce, and my older brother was in high school, and I didn't really know him. I did have friends, but everyone thought I was weird and to be honest, if weird means being different, I was weird. When I saw butterflies, I used to dance with them, and then when I saw chipmunks, I used to speak to them and tell them that I hoped they were having a wonderful day. The other kids laughed and said I was weird. I thought so, too. Kinda, but that's not the bullying. I was teased for wearing oversized clothes. I was heavier than the other girls in my class, and after we saw a documentary on African animals, the kids called me "hippo." My situation was made worse by early puberty, and I expanded everywhere. I was even bigger than I had ever been.

"The mean girls got really mean then. It was particularly bad at recess and at gym. I could not keep up with anyone, and the girls started to say they should have a "hippo race." At lunch, they commented on everything I ate. "Hippos have big mouths," they said making grunting sounds. Even my friends eventually looked away. No one stood up for me. Once in class, someone slipped me a note that said that there was an opening for hippos at our zoo.

"When I got home after school every day, I just did my homework, but I was crying inside. I saw my mom crying cause of the divorce, so I didn't tell her what had happened at school. I still had some friends, and they were great when they came to my house but at school they never stood up against the mean girls. I like to think that I would have done things differently if I were them, but would I? So, if your friends won't stick up for you, and your parents are too distracted, and your older brother has his own life, how do you stick up for yourself? But eventually, I could

not take it anymore and I told my mom and she cried, but I think that she was crying for herself. She told me that they would take me out of that school and put me in a private school. I felt so relieved, but to be honest, the names carried on there. Not as bad as in the public school, but still I heard what people said. With my weight and the bullying and my parents' divorce, I was the common denominator. No one else was to blame. Clearly, I was a terrible human being, and so I joined them and I started to hate myself, and use all the negative terms that others had used toward me, on myself. I made the problem worse. I started purging and restricting. My weight went all over the place. So, now I had an eating disorder. I was the common denominator.

"But then you asked me how I had learned to hate myself, and the question threw me for a loop. Had I learned to hate myself? Could I learn not to? Had all these terrible experiences taught me something that no one had corrected?

"I started to pay attention to my true self, separating my dreams and aspirations of today, from my early childhood experiences. Why did it take me so long to realize that I am not defined by the opinions of others, especially the ones who had never cared for me? Was it possible for me to learn that I have some value and maybe that I am worthy of love? Including from myself? But who determines that other than me? Once I got that, I started to work on dismantling all the pillars of self-hatred. The ones that had propped me up. I started to spend more time doing what brought me joy. I gave up my administrator position and went back to school for mental health counseling. I liked the people around me and they seemed to like me. I defined myself more through my relationship with them, rather than those 5th grade girls. And so here I am, not perfect by any means, OK as I am, and working every day to be more OKer ... is that even a word?"

These are powerful words indeed. All stories shared throughout this book are a testament to the resilience and hope of those who, through hard work, have faced the painful darkness of self-hatred and emerged with renewed perspectives. These narratives capture the pain of self-hate as well as transformation, illustrating that even the most ingrained negative beliefs can be challenged and changed. No one does this overnight. Embarking on the journey from self-loathing to self-compassion is not a quick fix. It requires patience, persistence, and the willingness to confront deeply held beliefs.

Through various approaches shared in the lived experiences of my patients – whether it's redefining personal narratives, making conscious choices, or embracing a more accurate truth of who they are – each one has found ways to dismantle the pillars of self-hatred and build a foundation of self-respect and acceptance.

The journey toward self-compassion will be both deeply personal and deeply transformative. By utilizing the practices and ideas presented in this book, you will be taking on the steps necessary to move away from self-hatred to uncover the inherent worth and wonder within you. Embrace the small victories, each one counts. Celebrate your progress, it is all movement in the right direction. Every self-affirming action is one of self-kindness, and each one matters. The path will be difficult at times, but the destination is worth every step. You are not alone and you are worthy of the outcome.

Chapter 17

AI's Take on Self-Hatred

As we wrap up this book, I have a late addition to the writing and it's to see whether technology, and in particular Artificial Intelligence (AI) can help you overcome self-hatred. I don't think that the answer will surprise you.

I was talking to a patient about his use of AI to help him with his college essays. If you are not aware of artificial intelligence, AI is a very powerful and complex computer software technology that increasingly appears to act the way a human brain does. Today almost every major industry uses AI, and it has become so sophisticated and disruptive a technology, that in many situations it is nearly impossible to know whether an essay, a photo, a voice, a math equation, a design, and so on, was created by a human or an AI. My patient went on to show me examples of how AI works. *"By using an AI platform, you put in a prompt about anything, and the AI responds. If you want an essay on thirteenth century footwear, it will do that. If you want computer code for some math equation, it will do that, if you want to write quirky wedding vows, it will do that. Not only will the AI do so, but you might want quirky wedding vows in the writing style of William Shakespeare. AI will do that," he said.*

I decided to put AI to the test and used Google's AI known as Bard. I went to the Bard site at: https://bard.google.com/ and asked the question: "*What is self-hatred and how is it treated?*" Here is the answer verbatim and without any editing. This writing is NOT my own writing, but rather the "reflections," if we can call them reflections, of artificial intelligence.

Conquering the Shadow Within: Tools for Battling Self-Hatred

Self-hatred, a venomous shadow that creeps into our hearts, can distort our perception and cripple our progress. It's a heavy burden to bear, whispering negativity and painting our flaws in the starkest hues. But amidst this darkness, remember, the embers of self-compassion and acceptance still glow. Here, we explore tools to rekindle these embers and illuminate the path towards self-love.

Understanding the Source:

Self-hatred rarely arises in a vacuum. It's often the tangled consequence of past hurts, negative experiences, or unrealistic expectations. Recognizing the root of this self-criticism is crucial. Was it a critical upbringing, a past misstep, or societal pressures? Unraveling these threads can help dismantle the negativity's hold.

Challenging the Inner Critic:

Our inner critic can be a harsh judge, amplifying flaws and dwelling on failures. Counter its voice with reason and kindness. Ask yourself: "Would I speak to a loved one this way?" Challenge negative thoughts with evidence of your strengths and accomplishments. Remember, progress, not perfection, is the true measure of worth.

Practicing Self-Compassion:

Treat yourself with the same understanding and tenderness you'd extend to a dear friend. Forgive your shortcomings, acknowledge your struggles, and celebrate your victories, big or small. Self-compassion is the fertile ground where self-love blossoms.

Embracing Mindfulness:

The present moment holds immense power. When self-hatred's tide threatens to engulf you, practice mindfulness. Focus on your breath, bodily sensations, or the sights and sounds around you. Grounding yourself in the present detaches you from the whirlwind of negative thoughts and allows for calmer self-reflection.

Cultivating Gratitude:

Shifting your focus from what you lack to what you possess fosters appreciation and counters negativity. Practice gratitude journaling, taking time each day to acknowledge the blessings, big and small, that enrich your life. Gratitude unlocks a treasure trove of self-worth.

Seeking Support:

Remember, you're not alone in this battle. Sharing your struggles with a trusted friend, family member, therapist, or support group can provide invaluable solace and guidance. Their empathy and lived experiences can illuminate your path and remind you that you're worthy of love and support.

Remember, healing is a journey, not a destination. There will be stumbles and setbacks, but with every step of self-compassion and acceptance, the grip of self-hatred loosens. Embrace the tools mentioned above, and nurture the seeds of self-love within you. Slowly, steadily, the darkness will recede, and your inner light will shine brighter than ever before.

Beyond the Essay:

Remember, this essay is just a starting point. Your unique experiences and insights will shape your narrative, making it both powerful and impactful. Here are some additional prompts to consider:

- *Share a personal anecdote or story that exemplifies your struggles with self-hatred and the tools you used to overcome them.*
- *Explore the societal factors that contribute to self-hatred, such as unrealistic beauty standards or toxic masculinity.*
- *Discuss the link between self-hatred and mental health conditions like anxiety or depression.*
- *Offer words of encouragement and support to others battling self-hatred, emphasizing the possibility of healing and self-acceptance.*

By weaving your own story and experiences into this framework, you can create an essay that not only informs but also inspires and empowers others facing similar challenges. May your words become beacons of hope, guiding yourself and others towards the radiant shores of self-love.

I hope this helps!

I am very curious to know what you think of the above and whether AI is sophisticated enough, at this point in time, to answer these types of questions, questions about the person you are and about how to change core personality traits. To my ear, it sounds non-human in tone, non-empathic in understanding, predictable in its advice, and bizarre in its attempt to portray self-loathing in dramatic prose. And so, as of the time of the completion of this manuscript in late 2024, I do not think that AI has evolved to the point that it is a useful tool in combating self-loathing.

But might AI be able to help? Here is my take on an AI solution. Although AI is fundamentally changing many aspects of the human experience by, for instance, automating tasks, analyzing data, helping with health care diagnostics, improving transportation flow, recognizing human language, enhancing computer vision and so on, there is one thing that it will never be able to do. It will never actually feel.

Human emotions are a complex set of psychological and physiological responses, and neither software nor hardware have the consciousness nor biology that is necessary to feel. While AI programs can now detect and, in many cases, accurately respond to the facial and physiological changes that manifest with human emotions, they will never viscerally experience them. AI will learn to validate others' emotions, and the responses will often feel accurate, but AI will never know what it is to feel emotional pain. It will never understand what it is like to feel that it is such a burden that it feels that it should no longer exist. It will never know what it is like to experience suffering so enduring and unrelenting that it begins to contemplate suicide. There is no amount of logic that can make AI deeply feel the crippling effects of self-hatred.

Some may argue that most therapists will never feel the level of desperation that you feel, but different from any machine or computer program, therapists do experience feelings, including suffering. So, unless there is a massive technological advance, for the foreseeable future, your progress to healing from self-hatred should not depend on being truly understood by an AI.

Afterword

Self-hatred is not an insurmountable challenge. It is true that if you slow down and start and think about the magnitude of the journey ahead, that you might consider it an impossible task. If you are open to the idea that you can overcome it, you will overcome it. Whether the people who have hurt you remain in your life or not, you no longer have to nurture the damage done by believing their false narrative. Once you realize that most of what torments you are the falsehoods and untruths that you continue to focus on, you have the key to freedom from the pain of self-hatred. I would not have written this book had I not been witness to the successful healing of so many courageous people who dared to believe that their lives could be different. You've got this!

References

Chapter 1

American Psychiatric Association (2022). *Diagnostic and Statistical Manual of Mental Disorders* (5th ed., text rev.), American Psychiatric Association.

Beuchat, Hélène, Grandjean, Loris, Junod, Nastia, Despland, Jean-Nicolas, Pascual-Leone, Antonio, Martin-Sölch, Chantal, & Kramer, Ueli. (2023). Evaluation of expressed self-contempt in psychotherapy: an exploratory study, *Counselling Psychology Quarterly*, 10.1080/09515070.2023.2201417

Christensen, AJ, Moran, PJ, Ehlers, SL, Raichle, K, Karnell, L, Funk, G. (1999). Smoking and drinking behavior in patients with head and neck cancer: effects of behavioral self-blame and perceived control. *Journal of Behavioral Medicine* 1999 22(5):407–18. 10.1023/a:1018669222706. PMID: 10586379.

Glinder, Judith G., and Bruce E. Compas. (1999). "Self-blame attributions in women with newly diagnosed breast cancer: a prospective study of psychological adjustment." *Health Psychology* 18.5: 475.

Janoff-Bulman, R. (1979). Characterological versus behavioral self-blame: inquiries into depression and rape. *Journal of Personality and Social Psychology*, 37, 1798–1809.

Mongrain, M. (1998). "Parental representations and support-seeking behaviors related to dependency and self-criticism". *Journal of Personality* 66 (2): 151–173. 10.1111/1467-6494.00007. PMID 9529661.

Overton, P. G., Markland, F. E., Taggart, H. S., Bagshaw, G. L., and Simpson, J. (2008). Self-disgust mediates the relationship between dysfunctional cognitions and depressive symptomatology. *Emotion* 8, 379–385. 10.1037/1528-3542.8.3.379

Rüsch, N., Oexle, N., Thornicroft, G., Keller, J., Waller, C., Germann, I., Regelmann, C.A., Noll-Hussong, M. and Zahn, R. (2019). Self-contempt as a predictor of suicidality: a longitudinal study. *The Journal of Nervous and Mental Disease*, 207(12), pp.1056–1057.

Santor, D.A.; Pringle, J.D.; Israeli, A.L. (2000). "Enhancing and disrupting cooperative behavior in couples: effects of dependency and self-criticism following favorable and unfavorable performance feedback". *Cognitive Therapy and Research* 24 (4): 379–397. 10.1023/A:1005523602102. S2CID 3022781.

The Dalai Lama, H. H. (1999). *Ethics for the New Millennium*. New York: Riverhead Books

Voth, J, Sirois, FM. (2009). The role of self-blame and responsibility in adjustment to inflammatory bowel disease. *Rehabilitation Psychology* 54(1):99–108. 10.1037/a0014739. PMID: 19618709.

Ypsilanti, A, Gettings, R, Lazuras, L, Robson, A, Powell, PA, Overton, PG. (2020). Self-disgust is associated with loneliness, mental health difficulties, and eye-gaze avoidance in war veterans with PTSD. *Frontiers in Psychology* 11:559883. 10.3389/fpsyg.2020.559883. PMID: 33192823; PMCID: PMC7662446.

Chapter 2

Nilsson, M., Lundh, L. G., & Westling, S. (2022). Childhood maltreatment and self-hatred as distinguishing characteristics of psychiatric patients with self-harm: a comparison with clinical and healthy controls. *Clinical Psychology and Psychotherapy*, 29(5), 1778–1789.

Turnell, A. I., Fassnacht, D. B., Batterham, P. J., Calear, A. L., & Kyrios, M. (2019). The self-hate scale: development and validation of a brief measure and its relationship to suicidal ideation. *Journal of Affective Disorders*, 245, 779–787. https://doi.org/10.1016/j.jad.2018.11.047

Wilner, JG, Ronzio, B, Gillen, C, Aguirre, B. (2024). Self-hatred: the unaddressed symptom of borderline personality disorder. *Journal of Personality Disorders* 38(2):157–170. 10.1521/pedi.2024.38.2.157. PMID: 38592908.

Chapter 5

Sender, R., Fuchs, S., & Milo, R. (2016). Are we really vastly outnumbered? Revisiting the ratio of bacterial to host cells in humans. *Cell*, 164(3), 337–340.

Chapter 6

Ille, R., Schöggl, H., Kapfhammer, H. P., Arendasy, M., Sommer, M., & Schienle, A. (2014). Self-disgust in mental disorders—symptom-related or disorder-specific? *Comprehensive psychiatry*, *55*(4), 938–943.

Levy, S. T. (1984). Psychoanalytic perspectives on emptiness. *Journal of the American Psychoanalytic Association*, 32(2), 387–404.

Linehan, M. M. (1993). *Skills Training Manual for Treating Borderline Personality Disorder*. Guilford Press.

Mahler, Margaret & Pine, Fred & Bergman, Anni. (1975). The Psychological Birth of the Human Infant: Symbiosis and Individuation. 10.4324/9780429482915.

Singer, M. (1977). The experience of emptiness in narcissistic and borderline states: II. The struggle for a sense of self and the potential for suicide. *International Review of Psycho-Analysis*, *4*(4), 471–479.

Chapter 7

Calati, R., Bakhiyi, C. L., Artero, S., Ilgen, M., & Courtet, P. (2015). The impact of physical pain on suicidal thoughts and behaviors: Meta-analyses. *Journal of psychiatric research*, 71, 16–32.

Klonsky, E. D., & May, A. M. (2015). The three-step theory (3ST): A new theory of suicide rooted in the "ideation-to-action" framework. *International Journal of Cognitive Therapy*, *8*(2), 114–129.

Smith, AR, Ribeiro, JD, Mikolajewski, A, Taylor, J, Joiner, TE, Iacono, WG. (2012). An examination of environmental and genetic contributions to the determinants of suicidal behavior among male twins. *Psychiatry Research* 197(1–2):60-5. 10.1016/j.psychres.2012.01.010. Epub 2012 Mar 13. PMID: 22417928; PMCID: PMC3376176.

Van Orden, KA, Witte, TK, Cukrowicz, KC, Braithwaite, SR, Selby, EA, Joiner, TE Jr. (2010). The interpersonal theory of suicide. *Psychol Rev.* 117(2): 575–600. doi: 10.1037/a0018697. PMID: 20438238; PMCID: PMC3130348.

Chapter 8

Wilner, JG, Ronzio, B, Gillen, C, Aguirre, B. (2024). Self-hatred: the unaddressed symptom of borderline personality disorder. *Journal of Personality Disorders* 38(2):157–170. 10.1521/pedi.2024.38.2.157. PMID: 38592908.

Chapter 9

American Psychiatric Association. (2022). *Diagnostic and Statistical Manual of Mental Disorders*. (5th ed., text rev.) https://doi.org/10.1176/appi.books.9780890425787

Doron, G, Moulding, R, Kyrios, M, Nedeljkovic, M. (2008). Sensitivity of self-beliefs in obsessive compulsive disorder. *Depression and Anxiety*; 25(10): 874–84. 10.1002/da.20369. PMID: 18033729.

Fairchild, H, Cooper, M. (2010). A multidimensional measure of core beliefs relevant to eating disorders: preliminary development and validation. *Eating Behaviors* 11(4):239–46. 10.1016/j.eatbeh.2010.05.004. Epub 2010 May 31. PMID: 20850058

Khosravi, M. (2020). Eating disorders among patients with borderline personality disorder: understanding the prevalence and psychopathology. *Journal of Eating Disorders* 8, 38. https://doi.org/10.1186/s40337-020-00314-3

Petersson, S., Birgegård, A., Brudin, L. et al. (2021). Initial self-blame predicts eating disorder remission after 9 years. *Journal of Eating Disorders* 9, 81. https://doi.org/10.1186/s40337-021-00435-3

Chapter 10

Kowalchyk, M., Palmieri, H., Conte, E., & Wallisch, P. (2021). Narcissism through the lens of performative self-elevation. *Personality and Individual Differences*, 177, 110780.

Ma, J., Xiong, Y., & Zhang, Y. (2023). The impact of childhood abuse on adolescent school bullying: the chain-mediated effects of self-loathing and peer relationships. *International Journal of Frontiers in Sociology*. Vol. 5, Issue 12: 59–63. https://doi.org/10.25236/IJFS.2023.051210.

Otani, K, Suzuki, A, Matsumoto, Y, Shirata, T. (2018). Marked differences in core beliefs about self and others, between sociotropy and autonomy: personality vulnerabilities in the cognitive model of depression. *Neuropsychiatric Disease and Treatment* 27;14:863–866. 10.2147/NDT.S161541. PMID: 29628763; PMCID: PMC5877496.

Rozental, A., Forsström, D., Hussoon, A., & Klingsieck, K. B. (2022). Procrastination among university students: differentiating severe cases in need of support from less severe cases. *Frontiers in Psychology*, 13, 783570.

Chapter 11

Bateman, A., & Fonagy, P. (1999). Effectiveness of partial hospitalization in the treatment of borderline personality disorder: a randomized controlled trial. *American Journal of Psychiatry*, 156(10), 1563–1569.

Beck, A. T. (1987). Cognitive models of depression. *Journal of Cognitive Psychotherapy: An International Quarterly*, 1, 5–37

Drozek RP, Unruh BT. Mentalization-based treatment for a physician with borderline personality disorder. *American Journal of Psychotherapy* 2022 75(1):51–54. 10.1176/appi.psychotherapy.20210019. Epub 2022 Jan 12. PMID: 35016553.

Krawitz, R. (2012). Behavioural treatment of severe chronic self-loathing in people with borderline personality disorder. Part 2: self-compassion and other interventions. *Australasian Psychiatry*, 20(6), 501–506.

Leaviss, J, Uttley, L. (2015). Psychotherapeutic benefits of compassion-focused therapy: an early systematic review. *Psychological Medicine* 45(5):927–45. 10.1017/S0033291714002141. Epub 2014 Sep 12. PMID: 25215860; PMCID: PMC4413786.

Linehan, M. M. (1993). *Skills Training Manual for Treating Borderline Personality Disorder*. Guilford Press.

Neely, ME, Schallert, DL, Mohammed, SS, Roberts, RM, Chen, YJ (2009). Self-kindness when facing stress: the role of self-compassion, goal regulation, and support in college students' well-being. *Motivation and Emotion* 33, 88–97.

Neff, KD, Kirkpatrick, KL, Rude, SS. (2007). Self-compassion and adaptive psychological functioning. *Journal of Research in Personality* 41, 139–154.

Laura Sallin, Isabelle Geissbüehler, Loris Grandjean, Hélène Beuchat, Chantal Martin-Soelch, Antonio Pascual-Leone & Ueli Kramer (2021). Self-contempt, the working alliance and outcome in treatments for borderline personality disorder: an exploratory study. *Psychotherapy Research* 31:6, 765–777, 10.1080/10503307.2020.1849848

Van Dam, NT, Sheppard, SC, Forsyth, JP, Earleywine, M. (2011). Self-compassion is a better predictor than mindfulness of symptom severity and quality of life in mixed anxiety and depression. *Journal of Anxiety Disorders* 25, 123–130.

Chapter 15

American Psychiatric Association. (2022). *Diagnostic and Statistical Manual of Mental Disorders* (5th ed., text rev.) https://doi.org/10.1176/appi.books.9780890425787

Amiri, S., Mirfazeli, F.S., Grafman, J. et al. (2023). Alternation in functional connectivity within default mode network after psychodynamic psychotherapy in borderline personality disorder. *Annals of General Psychiatry* 22, 18. https://doi.org/10.1186/s12991-023-00449-y

Back, Sarah N.; Schmitz, Marius; Koenig, Julian; Zettl, Max; Kleindienst, Nikolaus; Herpertz, Sabine C. and Bertsch, Katja (2022): Reduced vagal activity in borderline personality disorder is unaffected by intranasal oxytocin administration, but predicted by the interaction between childhood trauma and attachment insecurity. In: *Journal of Neural Transmission*, Vol. 129, No. 4: pp. 409–419

Gadeikis, D, Bos, N, Schweizer, S, Murphy, F, Dunn, B. (2017). Engaging in an experiential processing mode increases positive emotional response during recall of pleasant autobiographical memories. *Behaviour Research and Therapy* 92:68–76. 10.1016/j.brat.2017.02.005. Epub 2017 Feb 21. PMID: 28273505; PMCID: PMC5390771.

Gattuso, JJ, Perkins, D, Ruffell, S, Lawrence, AJ, Hoyer, D, Jacobson, LH, Timmermann, C, Castle, D, Rossell, SL, Downey, LA, Pagni, BA, Galvão-Coelho, NL, Nutt, D, Sarris, J. (2023). Default mode network modulation by psychedelics: a systematic review. *The International Journal of Neuropsychopharmacology* 26(3):155–188. 10.1093/ijnp/pyac074. PMID: 36272145; PMCID: PMC10032309.

Hafkemeijer, L, de Jongh, A, van der, Palen, J, Starrenburg, A. (2020). Eye movement desensitization and reprocessing (EMDR) in patients with a personality disorder. *European Journal of Psychotraumatology* 11(1):1838777. 10.1080/20008198.2020.1838777. PMID: 33425243; PMCID: PMC7755323.

Hauschildt, M, Peters, MJ, Moritz, S, Jelinek, L. (2011). Heart rate variability in response to affective scenes in posttraumatic stress disorder. *Biological Psychology* 88(2–3):215–22. 10.1016/j.biopsycho.2011.08.004. Epub 2011 Aug 19. PMID: 21856373.

Kähkönen, JE, Krämer, UM, Buades-Rotger, M, Beyer, F. (2021). Regulating interpersonal stress: the link between heart-rate variability, physical exercise and social perspective taking under stress. *Stress* 24(6):753–762. 10.1080/10253890.2021.1907339. Epub 2021 Apr 5. PMID: 33818287.

Kim, JJ, Parker, SL, Doty, JR, Cunnington, R, Gilbert, P, Kirby, JN. (2020). Neurophysiological and behavioural markers of compassion. *Scientific Reports* 10(1):6789. 10.1038/s41598-020-63846-3. PMID: 32322008; PMCID: PMC7176659.

Kop, WJ, Synowski, SJ, Newell, ME, Schmidt, LA, Waldstein, SR, Fox, NA. (2011). Autonomic nervous system reactivity to positive and negative mood induction: the role of acute psychological responses and frontal electrocortical activity. *Biological Psychology*. 86(3):230–8. 10.1016/j.biopsycho.2010.12.003. Epub 2010 Dec 21. PMID: 21182891; PMCID: PMC3061260.

Morton, E, Sakai, K, Ashtari, A, Pleet, M, Michalak, EE, Woolley, J. (2023). Risks and benefits of psilocybin use in people with bipolar disorder:

An international web-based survey on experiences of 'magic mushroom' consumption. *Journal of Psychopharmacology.* 37(1):49–60. 10.1177/02698811221131997. Epub 2022 Dec 14. PMID: 36515370; PMCID: PMC9834328.

Russell, ME, Scott, AB, Boggero, IA, Carlson, CR. (2017). Inclusion of a rest period in diaphragmatic breathing increases high frequency heart rate variability: implications for behavioral therapy. *Psychophysiology* 54(3): 358–365. 10.1111/psyp.12791. Epub 2016 Dec 7. PMID: 27925652; PMCID: PMC5319881.

Sheline, YI, Barch, DM, Price, JL, Rundle, MM, Vaishnavi, SN, Snyder, AZ, Mintun, MA, Wang, S, Coalson, RS, Raichle, ME. (2009). The default mode network and self-referential processes in depression. *Proceedings of the National Academy of Sciences of the United States of America.* 106(6): 1942–7. 10.1073/pnas.0812686106. Epub 2009 Jan 26. PMID: 19171889; PMCID: PMC2631078.

Tan, G, Dao, TK, Farmer, L, Sutherland, RJ, Gevirtz, R. (2011). Heart rate variability (HRV) and posttraumatic stress disorder (PTSD): a pilot study. *Applied Psychophysiology and Biofeedback* 36(1):27–35. 10.1007/s10484-010-9141-y. PMID: 20680439.

Weise, S, Parzer, P, Fürer, L, Zimmermann, R, Schmeck, K, Resch, F, Koenig, J (2020). Autonomic nervous system activity and dialectical behavioral therapy outcome in adolescent borderline personality pathology. *The World Journal of Biological Psychiatry.* https://doi.org/10.1080/.156229752020.1858155

I Hate Myself

TRIGGER WARNING: My goal is for this book to be a complete review of the topic of self-hatred. In this context, I dive into the scant research on the topic, but mostly I rely on, and am motivated by, the thoughtful reflections of the people who have shared their experiences with me. The accounts in this book are true disclosures of their experiences. They are the words of patients who have overcome, or are working on overcoming, self-loathing. They are honest about its impact on their lives. Some of them have been completely transparent about attempting suicide. Some of the accounts may trigger self-harm thoughts. They and I agree that suicide is not the answer to self-hatred, and that even when suicide thoughts creep back in, the focus remains on a life of purposeful living and intentional action. You will hear me say this throughout the book: Suicide is never the answer. I have not lived the life of my patients, and I cannot imagine their suffering, but they are a blessing in my life, and I find tremendous hope in the efforts that they have made to overcome their suffering. If you feel triggered by descriptions in the book, please contact your therapist or call the National Suicide Prevention Lifeline at 988.

Acknowledgments and Gratitude

I asked some patients who are new to me, and those who I have known for a long time, to help me figure out a way to change the experience of self-hatred. I had another big ask, that they be willing to challenge the idea that self-hatred is fixed and try some of the exercises I assigned. I accepted that they would be skeptical at times; however, that even at those times, that they would continue to practice the exercises, and then participate fully in both thought and action, whether skeptical or not, as if self-hatred can change.

More than for anyone else, this book is a dedication to their hard work, their shared insights, their honesty, and their fundamental love for others. I hope that the style of writing is helpful. In some sections it is a dialogue with my patients, in others, my own reflections, and in others yet a review of the existing literature. In alphabetical order, because you are all awesome and there is no hierarchy here, some of the contributors include: Annie R, Devon P, Fiona S, Grace G, Lauren W, MM, Roma D, and YT. Thank you for your courage and compassion that will resonate in unknown ways for countless people.

To Jewel, a kindred spirit and dear friend, thank you for challenging me to think beyond where I get to on my own!

For my son Anthony, for Kristen R, Kristen B, and Jessica P, all of whom worked with me on 3East, and Emma L who worked with me at Klarman, and Sarah L and Susan Z, two wonderful parents who reviewed the early chapters, thank you for reviewing and giving me such great feedback.

To Drs. Julianne Tirpak and Philip and Rebecca Resnik. Thank you for your ongoing research efforts in the area of self-hatred.

To Jed and Gillian, who let me crash at their place while life was complicated.

And finally, my team at Wiley. Tracy who introduced me to Leah. Leah who believed in the project and whose team came up with the title and cover, and for Emily, a brilliant editor who asked profound questions and pointed out the obvious when I missed it. Well not quite finally! I am so grateful to eagle-eyed copyeditor Debbie Williams who caught every inconsistent citation and formatting error.

About the Author

Blaise Aguirre, MD, is a child and adolescent psychiatrist, and an Assistant Professor of Psychiatry at Harvard Medical School. He is a trainer in, and specializes in, dialectical behavior therapy (DBT) as well as other treatments for borderline personality disorder and associated conditions. He is the founding medical director of 3East continuum of care, an array of programs for teens and young adults that uses DBT to target the symptoms of borderline personality disorder (BPD) and related conditions.

Dr. Aguirre has been a staff psychiatrist at McLean Hospital since 2000 and is nationally and internationally recognized for his extensive work in the treatment of mood and personality disorders in adolescents. He lectures regularly throughout the world. Dr. Aguirre is the author or co-author of multiple books, including *Borderline Personality Disorder in Adolescents*, *Mindfulness for Borderline Personality Disorder*, *Coping With BPD*, and the best-selling *DBT for Dummies*.

Index